James Haskell

PERFECT FIT
THE WINNING FORMULA

Transform your body in just 8 weeks
with my training and nutrition plan

HODDER &
STOUGHTON

First published in Great Britain in 2018
by Hodder & Stoughton
An Hachette UK company

3

Copyright © James Haskell 2018

A CIP catalogue record for this title is
available from the British Library

Trade Paperback ISBN: 978 1 473 64873 9
Ebook ISBN: 978 1 473 64874 6

Design and Art Direction: Smith & Gilmour
Photographer: Andrew Burton
Shoot Producer: Ruth Ferrier
Food Stylist: Emily Jonzen
Prop Stylist: Olivia Wardle
Performance Consultant: Jake Saunders
Models: Jake Saunders, Kirby Young, Tia Lewis
Equipment Supplier: Pulse Fitness
www.pulsefitness.com

Colour origination by Born Group

Printed and bound by Firmengruppe APPL,
aprinta druck, Wemding, Germany

Hodder & Stoughton policy is to use papers
that are natural, renewable and recyclable
products and made from wood grown in
sustainable forests. The logging and
manufacturing processes are expected to
conform to the environmental regulations
of the country of origin.

The information contained in this book is
not intended to replace the services of trained
health or fitness professionals or be a substitute
for medical advice. You are advised to consult
a doctor on any matters relating to your health,
and in particular on any matters that require
diagnosis or medical attention.

Hodder & Stoughton Ltd
Carmelite House
50 Victoria Embankment
London EC4Y 0DZ

www.hodder.co.uk

This book is for all the rugby fans and fitness
'keenos' who have supported me throughout my
career so far. Like you, I have always looked for
the answers on fitness and health. Hopefully my
book goes some way to helping you all start on
the right path, by cutting out all the nonsense.

CONTENTS

INTRODUCTION

Hello! Welcome to my book, and hopefully to the start of your new fitness journey. It's going to be fun, different and exciting. In an attempt to explain the best possible ways to fulfil your training goals, I have poured everything I have into this book. The result is a programme that can be shaped around you to find the perfect fit for your life. Within the pages of this book you will find the answers you are looking for, or at the very least some ideas on how to achieve your goals.

It's important to be honest from the start, so let's be clear – there are no miracles that will help you get into shape and change things for the better. You can spend your whole life searching for the holy grail of getting fit, which for most of us hopefully means doing nothing but still achieving good results. Sadly, despite what you might have read, watched or seen a celebrity endorse, you will never find that. You could eat vegetables till the cows come home, or coat yourself in firming gel while plugged into a muscle stimulation device, and all you will achieve is a sense of frustration and probably some health complications too.

That's really why I wrote this book – to cut through the nonsense, to break down the complications of the fad-ridden fitness world and to show that anyone can get in shape.

Before I started writing, I looked at other health and fitness books on the market, and was surprised by the sheer number available. All of them offered various ways of achieving those elusive healthy living and fitness goals, and some were really very good. Many, though, were written by people who have very little idea of what it actually takes to live a healthy life. Their authors claim to have gone from super-fat to super-in-shape by doing some very weird and wonderful things. There is no mention of the hours of personal training sessions they've had, or the dietary advice they've received. Instead they suggest that if you drink this, or do that for 10 minutes a day, you too will look like them.

This is rubbish and a dangerous yarn to spin. Aside from getting into shape once, a large number of those writers have never trained before or since, yet they are shaping the beliefs and actions of many trusting people. The fact is that those writers have been gifted with great genes, so they look like wonderful advertisements for their wacky claims. Or they got in shape once and spent the rest of the time photoshopping images of themselves.

Genetics play a huge role in terms of body shape and how people react to different nutrition and training stimuli. I have friends with the best bodies you could wish for, yet they eat take-aways every night of the week and show no adverse effects. It's galling for the rest of us, but we each have to live with our genetic inheritance.

My aim in writing *Perfect Fit* was to put everything I know to be truthful and proven about fitness into one book. What I advocate in these pages, I do myself every day. My training and nutrition record is here for everyone to see. I don't have formal qualifications yet, but they are being completed as you read this. What I do have, is 14 years experience of training, using trial and error to formulate the best results. This is what I am sharing with you.

Next time you see a reality TV star or somesuch talking about detox teas or being strong (when they clearly couldn't lift their own shopping, let alone a weight), remember to do your research before adopting their technique. If it seems too good to be true, that's exactly what it is.

This book looks at every aspect of what it takes to create the body you want and the healthy lifestyle that you deserve, and it does this thoroughly and systematically. I want you to imagine your pursuit of physical excellence as like creating a magnificent building: I am going to supply you with all the tools and materials to get this structure built. Every step you make and every little bit of progression is the equivalent of laying one more brick in the foundations of that structure. As you learn more and do more, you will be placing course upon course of bricks until you have built something you are proud of. The day you look in the mirror and see what you want is the day you place a flag of triumph on top of your building.

Through this process you will improve not just your body, but your physical and mental health, and your outlook on life. Remember, your brain is a muscle too, and also benefits from workouts. I know mine does.

When you come out the other side of *Perfect Fit*, you will understand what it takes to change your body. You will finally, I hope,

be able to see through the nonsense that bombards us every day in regard to nutrition, training, diet and self-help.

I firmly believe that if you want anything out of life, you must set yourself a goal, plan how you are going to get there, and put the work in to achieve it. You should never expect anything to be handed to you on a plate. And don't expect a magic pill or secret formula to get you into shape overnight. Like anything else that's worth achieving, it takes sacrifice, hard work and commitment.

Of course you will make mistakes and take knock-backs. I do every day of my life. The one thing that sticks with me always is something my father once said: 'You can lie to everyone else, but you can't lie to yourself.' I totally agree with that. Only you know whether you have done all it takes to be successful; only you will know if you've worked hard enough to get what you want. And please remember – hard work brings great rewards, in this case losing weight or gaining muscle and eating really good food.

I hope you will enjoy reading and using *Perfect Fit* as much as I enjoyed writing it. It's my hope that it will become your training and nutrition bible – something you will refer to as long as you have a desire for self-improvement.

LET ME INTRODUCE MYSELF

My name is James Haskell and I'm a professional rugby player for Wasps, England and the British and Irish Lions. I have been playing rugby across the world for the last 14 years, making over 200 appearances for Wasps, and 75 for England. I started my career in the UK, then moved to France, Japan, New Zealand and finally back to the UK. The teams I have played for on my world tour are:

>> Wasps
>> Stade Français
>> The Highlanders
>> Ricoh Black Rams

I have also had the opportunity to work my way through the England ranks from the England Under 18s to the full team. It was actually my failure to get into the England Under 16s that sparked my whole fitness journey, and is the reason behind writing this book. My national teams are:

>> England U18s, U19s, U21s
>> England 7s
>> England Saxons
>> England Senior Team
>> British & Irish Lions

Throughout my rugby career I have been lucky enough to work with the best in the business. That includes not just players, but also some of the world's premier trainers, conditioners, nutritionists and coaches. All these experiences have been distilled into my fitness philosophy, which will get you into shape not just for the short term, but for life.

For most people there is a catalyst that prompts them into adopting a fitter and healthier lifestyle. It could be a break-up, it could be health reasons, or, as in my case, a challenge. I was trialling for England Under 16s and got all the way to the final trial, but fell short. It was my first big disappointment and I didn't take it well.

One of the reasons for my failure was that I didn't do any of the suggested training. My father kept chasing me to train, but I did nothing except procrastinate. Frankly, I was unfit and did not have the size to compete in

the more high-profile games. It was a big ask at 14 to put some element of professionalism into my life, but I suppose that's what separates those who are committed from those who aren't. I certainly wasn't, and I chose going out with my friends and chasing girls over doing the extra fitness, strength and rugby work that would really have helped me.

I was so disappointed that I cried, and that's a big deal for a child who'd had a rather charmed life and always made the teams he aimed for. Of course I knew there were many bigger issues at stake in the world, but this was my first big reality check. It was the first time things hadn't gone my way. I felt very lost.

Nowadays in schools there is a culture of awarding participation medals, the idea being that taking part is just as good as winning. I think we all know that's rubbish. Life is not about taking part; it's a constant competition for jobs, partners and the lifestyle we individually want to have. If it weren't, we would all be millionaires and there would be no disappointment. I think we are doing the younger generation a disservice by mollycoddling them into thinking that they deserve awards just for turning up, and that mediocrity is acceptable. The simple truth is that if you want something worthwhile, you have to work for it, and this applies to getting a body you are comfortable with.

My dad told me I could take my failure to heart and give up on trying to play rugby any better than school level, or I could see it as a great opportunity to come back stronger. Even though I never actually wanted to be a rugby player, that challenge appealed to something fundamental in my personality – a burning desire to show people who doubt me that I can achieve what seems out of reach.

Luckily for me, a friend of the family – Henry Abrahamian – was a personal trainer, and he started coming into school twice a week for the last three years of my time at Wellington College. We would train from 9 to 10pm after I had finished my homework, and some afternoons after rugby practice. My priorities started to change, and instead of going out, I stayed in to train. While others chased girls, I was running up hills in the rain. I loved the idea of sacrificing to get what I ultimately wanted – results.

I became addicted to training, and the obsession developed over time to where I am now. Like a Rocky-style montage, I got fitter, bigger and more committed to what I was doing. I then trialled for England Under 18s and got in. It proved to me that hard work and dedication got results. If you want something, you have to sacrifice and work hard, it's that simple.

However, I wasn't happy with getting into just one team – I wanted more. I wanted to be in the best possible shape and be the best rugby player that I could. A little voice developed in my head that constantly questioned everything I did. It would say, 'Relax, take it easy, don't train, you'll be fine.' Quitting and resting are the easiest things to do, so whenever I heard the voice, I wanted to do the opposite. I found that the voice could drive me into pushing myself. This would often mean not drinking or eating what I wanted. If I did give in to temptation, I would train harder the next day to compensate. I never let up. If I was given fitness training to do, I would always find a place to do it, even on holiday in the most remote areas. I look back now and wonder what the hell I was doing.

Later on in my career I learnt to find a balance, and sometimes listened to the voice when it told me to rest. You need to be sensible about what you are doing and get the level right. That said, I still push the envelope and look into how I can improve.

Where fitness and diet are concerned, there is probably nothing I haven't tried or looked into. I believe you have to look around and find the best in the business to learn from, or try new things for periods of time to get those little percentage gains here and there. It doesn't do to be complacent about what's on offer. For example, it's often assumed that professional rugby clubs or national teams have the best coaches and managers, but I have not always found this to be the case. I learnt very early on that it's important to get a second opinion or to seek outside support across everything you are doing, whether that is fitness, nutrition, physio or medical care. You get only one shot at your career, and it would be a nightmare to look back and realise you didn't do all you could to get the best possible results.

Inevitably, this approach requires you to be single-minded, and I have been accused many times of being selfish. But as a sportsman, I believe you have to be selfish if you have only a short period of time in which to find success. The same approach is necessary if you want to get into the best possible shape and make progress in your life. Nobody cares more about the results you get than you do. Looking to others to have your best interests at heart is a fool's errand. As a result, I have always spent my own money in seeking out the best nutritionists, physiologists, trainers and coaches to help me on my way.

All the training I have ever undertaken has been done under the strictest rules. Even from an early age, I have been subject to WADA

(World Anti-Doping Agency) drug testing. This agency is often mentioned in the media, especially when it comes to the Olympics or the Tour de France, as it handles all the drug testing for professional sport around the world. Their scrutiny means you can be confident that everything I have achieved with my physique has been done naturally, safely and healthily. Oh, and without the help of Photoshopped images, unlike some Instagram celebs who promote their amazing lives and physiques online.

I tell you this because it's important that you know what is and isn't possible. You will always find doubters who feel that the achievements they witness are the result of trickery, cheating or quick fixes. Such people look past the hard work, sacrifice and pain that are the real reasons behind others' success. Trust me, if I can do it with the limited ability and talent I have, then imagine what you, the reader, can do with some direction and motivation. That is what I hope you will find within the pages of *Perfect Fit*.

THE CURRENT STATE OF PLAY

Having told you a little about where I came from, it's now time to tell you what I am doing now. Well, I am 32 and currently playing within the Aviva Premiership for Wasps. Also, when selected, I play for the England national team.

I have no desire to retire anytime soon, so all the lessons and advice I give within these pages are part of the regime I am still following myself every day. I've noticed that lots of coaches and trainers tend to have a

'Do as I say, not as I do' approach. They are normally the ones who post pictures of themselves always in shape and never admit to having bad days. My philosophy is 'Do as I say and do what I do'. In other words, I practise what I preach. You'll see this if you follow my social media channels, where I have shown my own transformation from holiday blob to something resembling a professional rugby player again.

Other than playing rugby, which takes up most of my time, I do motivational speaking, after-dinner speaking and DJing. But the most important sideline is my fitness business, James Haskell Health and Fitness. It was born about six years ago while I was playing rugby in New Zealand for the Highlanders.

The fitness business came about through the time I spent on Twitter and other social media channels, which at first I never really used for anything positive. It was only after I started posting a little about my daily routine – what I was eating, what kind of training I did, my views on certain products – plus the occasional photo of food and maybe a topless selfie (it was before 'selfie' was even a word) and bang! I suddenly got inundated with messages and follows.

I was amazed how much fans wanted to know what I was eating, what training I was doing, what my mentality was. I started to share information, which got an insane number of views, and I eventually realised that there were bigger things afoot. That's when I decided to create my fitness business, initially called JH BodyFire. It was a simple concept to start with, sharing a blog or two a week on what I had been doing and eating. I created the website myself using a free Google tool, and it went from there.

It took me a while to work out what direction I was going in. I think this is the same for everyone starting out with their own business. You think you have a plan and then, over time, everything changes. I was covering every topic, and working with every Tom, Dick and Harry to create content and posts.

My message was very mixed, and while I was pleased with all the content I put out, it wasn't clear exactly where I was hanging my hat. Was it fat loss, women's fitness, rugby, bodybuilding, UFC (Ultimate Fighting Championships) or something similar? All these topics are interests of mine, but they didn't really cohere.

I decided to focus on what I knew best – rugby and building muscle. This gave my business the direction it needed, and I have now come full circle after the success of my rugby training guide for men and women, *Becoming and Remaining Rugby Fit*, and my 12-week plan *The Lean Gains Bodybuilding Guide*, to write a book on general health and getting in shape. Everything I have ever done has been about sharing professional advice and tailoring it to every level of ability.

I wanted to share the book on rugby and pure muscle building first because sport and being match fit are my bread and butter. It was only when I looked around and saw there was huge demand for simple training and nutrition advice that I decided to go mainstream with what I was doing.

I have not reinvented training or created my own method of doing things. What I have done instead is to take the knowledge I have gleaned from the last 14 years of working with amazing 'gurus' and written it in such a way that even those with no experience at all of training and nutrition can get into shape. Of course I put my own spin on things, but that's the point of this book. There is really nothing new you need to know, other than what is already out there, but I think much of what has been written, explained and executed is simply wrong. I want to be your guide through the maze of the fitness world. I want to cut out the background noise and give you information straight from the horse's mouth. Yes, there are different ways of doing things, and new ways are created all the time, but some ways are the best.

So the book *Perfect Fit* was born! The ultimate guide for everyone from beginners to advanced trainers to get their body the way they want.

I HAVE NOT REINVENTED TRAINING OR CREATED MY OWN METHOD OF DOING THINGS. WHAT I HAVE DONE INSTEAD IS TO TAKE THE KNOWLEDGE I HAVE GLEANED FROM THE LAST 14 YEARS OF WORKING WITH AMAZING 'GURUS' AND WRITTEN IT IN SUCH A WAY THAT EVEN THOSE WITH NO EXPERIENCE AT ALL OF TRAINING AND NUTRITION CAN GET INTO SHAPE.

HOW TO USE THIS BOOK

I strongly recommend that you read this book from cover to cover in order to get the fullest picture of what's on offer. Chapter 1 contains all the general information you need to make some informed choices about tackling your shape and fitness issues. It tells you what to expect, how to set goals and the best way to avoid training pitfalls. This is followed by a chapter on pre-training advice – hints, tips and ideas for getting the most out of your training routine.

The core of this book is Chapter 3, which is devoted to the training programmes. The beginner's 8-week plan can be done at home without the use of gym. The idea is to help those who have never trained before to get used to moving and working out. It's also the place to start if you're not certain about your level of fitness or are very overweight. Perhaps most importantly, the 8-week programme is ideal for busy people because the training sessions are short and sharp, easy to slot into a packed day.

The beginner's plan is followed by the 12-week programme, which builds from medium intensity to high intensity, then a down week, followed by an increase in training intensity once again. It covers every day of the week and details how to lift properly and work out safely. The programme is set up in such a way that you can tailor it to your particular goal, whether that is weight loss, weight loss with muscle gain, or just pure muscle building. The plan is completely unisex, but in a few instances I have included some exercise options just for women because they don't usually want huge chests (well, not normally).

The alternative exercises are indicated in grey type within the programme are also there for those of you who may not have access to certain equipment, or who may need a simpler alternative. It's up to the user whether to do them or not.

All the exercises used in the training plans appear in Chapter 4. They are arranged in alphabetical order for ease of reference, and accompanied by fantastic photographs. You will never need to wonder if you are doing something correctly because you will have really clear references at your fingertips.

Chapter 5 deals with recovery, rest and mobility, which are massively important. They will help you to recover from the tough workouts, ensuring you are physically up to each day's challenges and able to achieve the results you are after.

As I am at pains to say throughout, training and diet go hand in hand, so Chapter 6 is devoted to nutrition. It explains calorie counting, macros and supplements, the carbohydrate meals you should be eating if you wish to gain size, and the protein-focused meals if you wish to lose weight. This will help you to build your personal diet plan.

The final chapters of the book are devoted to recipes, suggested meal plans and frequently asked questions. All in all, you now have everything you need to get training properly.

Twitter: @jameshaskell
Facebook: jameshaskelljhhf
Instagram: @jameshask
YouTube: thejameshaskell

Chapter 1
FITNESS AND YOU

Let's get this straight from the start. I have no miracle solutions or weird and wonderful things to sell. Neither do I have any cool slogans or catchphrases, such as 'Bosh!' or 'Guilty'. To be honest, I am a bit jealous I don't have one, so please feel to tweet me your ideas @jameshaskell.

What I am about is simple, direct and clear information about quality nutrition allied to a ferocious work ethic. I want to take people through a step-by-step routine to expand, develop and adjust their thinking about diet and training methods, and maybe even help with some life goals.

What I have learnt about training and getting into shape is that you need to train smart, have a plan, stay focused and be prepared to work. One size does not fit everyone, and at some stage you need to personalise what you are doing, yet you can still make amazing progress by following certain simple steps that will work for anyone. Furthermore, you don't need to spend thousands on blood tests, nutritionists, equipment and trainers to get into shape. Of course, if you *are* a professional sports person or looking to become a body competitor, I would advise taking these things to the next level. Otherwise, anyone can use this book and benefit from it. The only people who might need specialist treatment or advice are vegans, those with aggressive food allergies, and those who have serious diseases or ailments. *In all these cases, please check with your GP before embarking on the programme.*

I am neither a fitness guru nor a qualified training expert (yet), and there are many out there who know far more about these things than I do. What I am, however, is a person who has devoted his life to being in shape. There are any number of armchair pundits on social media – who just post something about fitness or health and watch the advice flood in – but I have got out of my armchair and put things into practice. That makes a world of difference.

Like everyone, I have changed my views over the years. That's the thing with diet and nutrition; it's not an exact science, and what is in vogue one day might be passé the next. You have to be prepared to put your hands up and say, 'I have changed my opinion about X, and I believe Y is now correct.'

Of course, the fundamentals never change, so it remains true that hard training and a clever nutrition plan will get you results. That is how you change your body. I have been living this lifestyle for 14 years and know how to change my shape.

What I am certain about is that *Perfect Fit* will help 95 per cent of you to be happy with what you see in the mirror. It will clear a path through the tangle of information that is the health and fitness world.

COMMON CONCERNS

'What's the best way to lose fat and build muscle?' 'How do I tone up?' 'Should women train differently from men?' 'Is it a good idea to juice?' 'Should I eat carbs' 'Can I train without using a gym?' 'Should I train fasted?'

These are just a tiny proportion of the questions that are currently being pinged around the world. To be honest, most of these came straight out of my various social media inboxes in one day. The questions reflect the fact that the fitness industry is very confusing. Everyone is working an angle and selling you a dream.

Why am I different? Because everything I recommend I have done myself. It's simple, fun, effective training and nutrition that will get you results. The only limiting factor is how hard are you prepared to work.

People, of course, are often lazy and looking for quick fixes. 'Can I eat what I want and still get fit?' 'Can I train only 10 minutes a day and still get in shape?' 'If I attach these electrodes to my stomach, will I get a six-pack?' The honest answer to all these questions is 'No'. Short cuts don't work. In fact, I shudder when I see adverts for abdominal electrodes. Who on earth thinks they are going to work?

The only way you are going to get into shape is through hard work and eating well. This will take as long as it takes. Some people will find it super-easy; others won't.

The 12-week training plan (see page 58) is designed for those of you who might have trained before, but have failed to get the results you want. It aims to bring together all the different advice you have been given in the past and tie it into one programme so you can finally get results. It will help you to get started, or kick-started if you've stopped, and give you a realistic goal. **However, complete beginners can start with the 8-week plan (see page 46), which can be done at home if you find public gyms intimidating.** It will teach you the basics so that when you progress to lifting weights, you will know what you should be doing. In my experience, a large number of young people want to dive straight into training, so the 8-week plan will help you to get results without starting on the weights too early.

Both the 8-week and the 12-week training plans are fun and provide a solid foundation, something you can revisit time and again, whenever you want to make improvements.

As with most things in life, the longer you follow your chosen plan, the better you will look. I feel the best results are achieved over 24 months, or even longer. After that period, I suggest you move your focus to another goal, perhaps strength or general fitness. I mention in this book the importance of not trying to be big, ripped, strong, fast and powerful all in one go. You need to split what you are doing into different goals and go after them individually. Unless you are genetically blessed or a freak, you can't achieve them all at once. After 24 months or whatever amount of time it takes until you feel happy with what you see in the mirror, I recommend you change up your goal and do another 12-week hit. Of course, you can stick with the programme for as long as you want, but your body needs a different stimulus to keep getting results. You can't do the same thing forever and expect to keep improving.

The plans I have written are put together in such a way that you can use them differently to achieve your own personal goal, which is probably one of the following:

» Weight loss
» Weight loss and muscle building
» Pure muscle building

My aim in this book has been to make the training programmes accessible to everyone. You will therefore be glad to hear that both the 8-week and the 12-week plans are the same for both sexes. Essentially, men and women will be doing the same thing at home, in the gym and with their diets.

'Why is it not different for women?' I hear you demand. 'Surely it should be.' The answer is that only clever marketing has made you think that women must train and eat differently from men. (I discuss this in more detail later.)

This book gives professional advice tailored to whatever level you might be at. It will help beginners to get started, while also helping others to improve and achieve the goals that might have seemed unattainable before.

HOW CAN I HELP?

My role is not so much about how I can help you; it's more about how I can guide you to help yourself. It's one thing to focus on fat loss alone – in fact, it's not that hard to drop some unwanted padding – but I want to offer you more than that. I want to get you into the best shape you can possibly be, whether that is lighter, heavier, more muscly or more defined.

I also want to teach you some fitness and nutrition lessons for life, lessons that you can keep referring back to at any time so that you can make the body changes you want whenever you want. Once you have these tools in your locker, you won't have to buy another plan or mad recipe book ever again.

One thing I want to state straight away is that I have never been overly fat. I don't know that struggle, and I don't pretend to know how hard it is to be unhappy with what you see in the mirror. Don't get me wrong. I am constantly looking for self-improvement, and am very rarely content with my body image. That, sadly, is a by-product of having trained for so many years.

Yet dissatisfaction has never been a defining factor of my everyday life. I have eaten myself out of shape a few times, most recently after I had the big toe on my left foot reconstructed. I went from 117kg to 124kg, and 10 per cent body fat to 18 per cent. For me, this was the equivalent of massively falling off the wagon.

I know a lot of you are probably thinking it's far from easy to make the changes I talk about, but trust me – **if you stick with the plan and put in the work, you *will* get results**. In fact, I want you to demand results *now*, and not be content with letting days go by without working to change your body image.

THE IMPORTANCE OF GOALS

My own reasons for training have simply been to achieve the goal of being in the healthiest shape I can. What drives me are results, not any battle against past demons. Yes, of course there is an element of vanity with wanting to look good, but if you don't already have some desire to look and feel better, you would never have picked up this book.

Like most readers of *Perfect Fit*, I have various things I would like to achieve in my life. The secret to achieving them is setting yourself small attainable goals that you can easily tick off. They need to be clearly defined and you need to focus on them 100 per cent. Say, for example, you want to be bigger, stronger, faster, fitter and more powerful. You have to fix on just one thing and go after it with all your might. Trying to achieve everything in one go is where many people fall down. The goals may be so varied that they end up working against each other, and the final result is failure.

It doesn't matter what your goal is, but make it clear and be realistic. I have read

The Secret and all manner of other self-help books that encourage you to ask the universe for help in being whatever you want, and they promise it will be delivered. With health and fitness, some things are more possible than others. There are many limiting factors that I will go into a bit later, but one at a time. The principal programme here is 12 weeks long, so you need to be level-headed about what your goal is going to be. Find it and stick to it.

When I suggested writing this programme, I was told that 12 weeks was too long a time, and that people want quicker progress and quicker fixes. However, to get the body you want – and I'm talking fitness, not just losing weight – 12 weeks is about the shortest time possible to get those insane results we all crave. You can of course start to see things change from 2–4 weeks, but in 12 weeks you will be blown away by what you see. I am sure those super-keenos amongst you could do things more quickly, but for most people 12 weeks is the perfect commitment span. It's long enough to get some amazing results, but I also think it will energise you to go on for much longer.

I firmly believe that as long as you are engaged and moving forward, you are achieving. Stagnation and comfort are signs that your momentum has stopped. **If you become casual about your goals, you will become a casualty to progress.** The same applies when it comes to getting into shape. If you are constantly doing the same thing day in, day out in the gym, or eating the same boring foods, your progress will drop off. You need to refresh what you are doing in order to maintain interest and progress.

It's important to remain hungry for self-improvement. The only time you stop learning or getting better is when you have drawn your last breath and left this mortal sphere. While you are alive and kicking, you can always do better and always improve.

Perfect Fit is set up in such a way that it will cater for whatever your initial goals might be. If you want to lose weight, it can help. If you want to build muscle and get ripped, it can sort that. At its simplest, the programme can just help to make you feel more confident about wearing a swimsuit.

I believe that life is for living and for being enjoyed, so I want to help you find a lifestyle that fits you as an individual. That is the secret of *Perfect Fit* – you can make it your own programme to fit your needs. It is not a diet: it's a nutrition plan and a way of life that allows you to eat well and enjoy your food. However, you can't escape the fact that if you want results, you have to put in the work. Some people will go full metal jacket on this programme and see it through, while others will do the bare minimum and not get what they want. Only you know which one of those you are going to be.

SO WHAT ARE YOUR GOALS?

We are all different, so our hopes and dreams, along with our training and dietary needs, are different too. What I want to achieve with my body, and my reasons for trying to get those results, are very different from someone else's, even in the rugby world. Yet the path to getting there and what you need to do when it comes to training and nutrition are very similar.

When I talk about having goals, what do I actually mean? Let me tell you some of the big, long-term targets that I'm currently aiming for.

» Keep playing rugby for Wasps and winning silverware.

» Play for England until the next World Cup, and be the best player in my position.

» Run my fitness business in such a way that I am constantly helping new people.

» Create the best range of tested sports supplements on the market.

» Keep learning and getting better every day by small margins of improvement.

» Have a bestselling range of fitness books that people use as training bibles.

» Remain in the best possible physical shape I can, which includes a heavy focus on my mobility.

» Reduce body fat in six weeks by 2 per cent.

» Commit to extra rugby skills for 10 minutes every day after training.

» Take Sunday off to prepare my food for the week.

These short-term goals are easily achievable and can be ticked off every day. They give a sense of progression and make sure I get stuff done.

KEEP TRACK OF YOUR GOALS

It's great to see both your short-term and long-term goals written down because it makes them feel real. That's why I have provided the charts opposite. You'll see that they already include some of the key elements you should focus on, but there is lots of space for you to fill in your own personal goals. Photocopy these charts and put them somewhere, such as on the fridge door, where they will spur you on to achieve success.

MAKING MISTAKES

We all fail sometimes, and we all make mistakes. Anyone who says they don't is lying. I always say to beware of boasters and remember to take their claims of having a perfect life with a pinch of salt. Only trust those who are open about their background and whom you know to be honest with their followers in life and on social media.

If you fail to hit a target or you come off your diet for a day, don't lose your head. It doesn't mean you have failed, and it doesn't mean you have to stop the programme. Just pick yourself up and go again. If you eat an unhealthy meal, it's not going to end all your progress, but eating five unhealthy meals in a row is a different matter.

Inevitably, these are very different from the kind of goals *you* need to be setting yourself. The point is that long-term goals should sit alongside your short-term fitness goal. They are not necessarily tangible or completely within your control, but they act like triggers or constant reminders that you can think about every day, and will help to steer how you think, train, eat and act. They take time to come to fruition, but they give me guidance in my daily life. If you have never thought about making a list of long-term goals, I strongly suggest you do.

I set far simpler short-term goals, such as:

Long-term goals

	3 months	6 months	1 year	3 years	5 years
Body shape					
Career					
Personal life					
Finance					
Travel plans					
Future job					
Qualifications					

Short-term goals

	Mon	Tues	Weds	Thurs	Fri	Sat	Sun
Week 1							
Week 2							
Week 3							
Week 4							
Week 5							
Week 6							
Week 7							
Week 8							
Week 9							
Week 10							
Week 11							
Week 12							

I struggle a lot with making mistakes in games, and it was my sports physiologist who came up with the idea that I should think of myself as an artist, and my goal (a great performance) as a painting. You don't just walk up to the canvas and get things perfect straight away. You make preliminary sketches, you make mistakes, which you crumple up and throw away. An artist's studio is littered with mistakes, and it's only in the gallery that you see the final article. Remember that failures are just attempts at aiming for the perfect outcome. It's better to try, make a mistake, regroup and go again, than never to try so that you never fail.

WHAT RESULTS CAN YOU EXPECT FROM THIS BOOK?

The one thing that everyone wants to know is what results to expect after following my plan for either 8 or 12 weeks. The simple answer is that if you follow all the information held within these pages, you will get some pretty amazing results. I give you my word on that.

Each of you will be starting your training at a different level, so that will affect how quickly things happen. Funnily enough, those of you who are super-overweight will see changes more quickly than others. Stick to the programme, though, and everyone will lose fat, gain muscle and look better in swimwear than you ever thought possible. It will take time, but it will happen. It's important you demand results, as this will push you on.

You might not end up with a physique like a *Men's Health* cover model, mine or Gigi Hadid's – that may not even be your inspiration – but you can end up looking better than you ever imagined. Just remember, though, there are a number of factors that will limit what kind of results you will get. Let's look at these in turn.

Time

Like everything in life, getting results takes time. What you put into this programme will reflect how much you get out of it, but it can take varying amounts of time for different people to get into shape. Some will find it easy, while others will need to work longer and harder to reach the same point. While I feel 12 weeks is the optimum amount of time to get some really potent results, I have also created a beginner's 8-week plan for those who want to build a base before embarking on the full 12-week programme.

For example, you can follow the 8-week plan to get used to training and burn some fat, then start the 12-week plan to focus on muscular development.

Effort

It's very simple: either you will work hard or you will cut corners. I won't be there to shout over your shoulder when you need it. This programme is as much a mental test as a physical one. Some of you will purchase this book, do the bare minimum or give up early and not get the results you want. You will then move on to the next plan and the cycle will continue. Some of you will do this plan to the letter; you will live and breathe it. These people will change their lifestyle, not just their training programmes or diet. They are testament to the fact that getting into shape takes effort and willpower, but it can still be fun. If all the good things in life, like being in shape and earning loads of money, were easy, we would all be doing it.

BODY TYPES

Both men and women fall into one of the following three categories of body type.

》Ectomorphs have a fast metabolism and do not gain muscle or fat easily. They require a high daily calorie intake with both high-carbohydrate and high-fat macros (see page 207) to build muscle.

》Mesomorphs have a moderate metabolism, building muscle relatively easily while remaining fairly lean, although they can gain excess body fat if consuming excess calories. They require a moderate daily calorie intake and tend to gain more muscle mass when consuming higher carb/lower fat macros (see page 207).

》Endomorphs have a slow metabolism, building muscle easily but also storing excess calories as fat. They require a lower daily calorie intake and tend to store less body fat when consuming slightly higher fat/lower carb macros. This nutritional information is all explained in more detail in Chapter 6.

FEMALE BODY SHAPES

》Rectangle is the most common body shape for women, accounting for around 46 per cent of the female population. Those who have this body shape carry weight proportionately and have a slim figure overall. Weight tends to be gained around the midsection or hips.

》Inverted triangle body shape accounts for around 14 per cent of women. The shoulders are wider than the hips, and the legs are often thin.

》Pear shape accounts for around 20 per cent of women. Those with this body shape have a slim waist and narrow shoulders compared to their hips and thighs.

》Hourglass body shape accounts for around 8 per cent of women. Weight is distributed evenly between the bust, upper arms, hips and thighs. Those with an hourglass shape maintain a tapered waist.

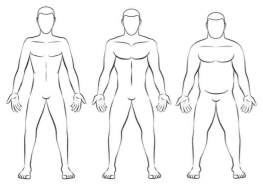

| Ectomorphs | Mesomorphs | Endomorphs |

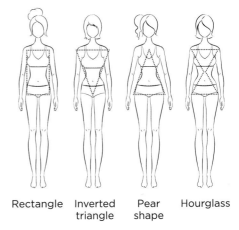

| Rectangle | Inverted triangle | Pear shape | Hourglass |

Genes

The last limiting factor, and one you can't do anything about, is your genetic inheritance. **You will either have a predisposition to be in shape and retain low body fat, or you will be the complete opposite. Your natural body shape plays a huge role in what you will achieve, and understanding this will help you get to grips with your rate of progress.** You might look great after just 6 weeks, or need more than 12 weeks to achieve your goal.

While it is true that women fit into the categories on the previous page, there are other shape descriptions that apply to them too. This is because women naturally retain far more body fat than men and need those extra deposits. In fact, it is dangerous for women to go below a certain body fat percentage.

Now you understand a little more about what is and isn't possible, it's important to keep perspective on what results you can expect. For example, I would love to have the body of The Rock or John Cena, but I don't take large amounts of special supplements and I can't train like them because they are wrestlers and I am a performance athlete who needs to peak every week to play a game.

Bear in mind too that if your starting point is way down the grid and you haven't seen your feet in two years, 12 weeks on my programme will not suddenly turn you into a health magazine cover model. It doesn't work like that. However, everything is possible over an extended period of time and eventually you can look like you have stepped from the pages of *Sports Illustrated*.

MISINFORMATION

I often sit at my computer going through my social media messages or reading the press, and end up with my head in my hands. There are so many mistakes, stupid suggestions and insane product promotions out there. The mind boggles as to where they all come from. My guess is that they stem from a desire to make cash, and those looking for a quick fix are easy prey.

Now let's be clear. For the most part, it's not the public's fault if they believe that something they read is true. The real problem lies with the media who perpetuate bad information, and with those in authority who fail to give good fitness and nutrition advice.

If you actually lived your life according to the conflicting reports you read or watch, you would know that red wine is one day good for you and bad for you the next; that broccoli apparently cures cancer but then is said to cause it; that fat is a no-no, yet is indisputably needed in our diet. Cereals and breakfast bars have also fluctuated in favour, praised for being fortified with vitamins, then rubbished for being full of sugar. Is it any wonder we're in a quandary about what to eat for optimum health?

I find that when I answer one question on social media and explain that you can't turn fat into muscle, nor can you tone up (whatever that means) by running on the pavement, another one will spring up in its place. It's a bit like plugging a hole in the side of a ship with your finger. Just as you stop it, another leak bursts out, so you use another finger. You end up with all your fingers and toes plugging leaks, yet more keep coming. That's essentially why I wrote this book. It's my mega leak stopper.

Of course, it's not just the mainstream media filling people's heads with rubbish. It's also the Instagram celebrities, online gurus and keyboard warriors, who do just as much damage. All you need is Google and no social life to suddenly start handing out fitness and health tips.

My first golden rule is not to believe everything you see online. I could take a photo of me standing next to a Ferrari and post it on Instagram with the caption, 'My new car', while I am actually driving around in my nan's Vauxhall Astra. Bogus information can undermine confidence and do a lot of damage.

The same principle applies to following fitness people online. False claims can throw you off your routine, undervalue your results and adversely affect your mindset. It takes a brave person to post a bad photo and tell you that they just seriously fell off their diet by eating a whole birthday cake. (This actually happened to me a few times after a tough training session at Wasps when I was younger, but that's a story for another day.)

There are of course some very reliable people out there who explain how things really work and post photos good and bad. It just takes time for the online user to winkle out the rubbish and find the genuine people. Some never do, and actually end up getting defrauded.

There is one online fraudster in particular who preys on unsuspecting victims looking to get in shape. I have no idea how he keeps getting away with it, but he takes your money and either fails to provide plans, or passes off others' plans as his own. More worryingly, he has also been known to recommend taking severe measures to get results, and these have massive health implications. He has been reported hundreds of times and there is plenty of online evidence unmasking his devious ways.

Yet people get caught up in his hype about all the 'transformations' he has to his name, and they blindly hand over the money. My advice is to do your research before entrusting someone with your money and health.

Another important point is to keep your body in perspective. Very few people are in shape all year round, and women also need to remember that they naturally carry more body fat than men – on average 6–11 per cent more. Studies have shown that the female hormone, oestrogen, burns fat more slowly than the male hormone, testosterone, and this results in more fat being stored around the body. The most likely reason, according to one study, is to prime women for childbearing. Whatever the reason, the outcome is that even women who look in shape still tend to have a higher body fat percentage than might be expected.

Like other men, I have been guilty of objectifying women and believing that they should look like lingerie models 24/7. Scrolling through Instagram or Twitter and seeing photos of people always looking 'hot' distorted my expectations. Now, though, since I have come to understand training and diet, my view has changed. I realise that nobody, except the very rare, are in shape all the time. People will do all sorts of things to prep for the photos they post, but the body condition they show the world will last 24–48 hours max. They will then have to rehydrate and refeed their depleted body, and consequently will stop looking superhuman.

'Hot bod' photos put the wrong expectations on men and women: they either feel they have to look a certain way, or start expecting other people to conform to that look. I learnt this the hard way. In my single days, a long, long time ago, I was chatting to a woman over Instagram. She had incredible pictures and looked the bomb. I assumed she always looked like her staged photos. It was only when we attended the same event and she came up to talk to me that I realised the truth. So marked was the difference between the photos and reality, I initially had no idea who she was, and it took five minutes of conversation to work out she was the woman on Instagram.

Getting information off the internet without doing your due diligence is like taking a car for a spin without having driven before. At some point you will crash, perhaps seriously. The moral is, don't be in a rush, do your research and you won't go wrong.

LADIES, LISTEN CLOSELY

There is so much rubbish written about women's fitness and the need for it to be different from men's. Yes, if you want to lose weight, you can't just do weights alone; you will to need to do more cardio than men do. It's also a fact that it's harder for women to build muscle, and the reason for that is a lack of testosterone. However, the process of building muscle is the same for both sexes; it just takes women longer.

Of course, women usually have different goals too. Men want big arms and six-packs, while women want flat stomachs and pert bottoms. You'll need to narrow your focus on these particular points, but to get your journey started, you all follow the same path.

Despite this, we are led to believe that women are a completely different species, needing special training programmes that are markedly different from men's. For the most part, women can do exactly the same as men to achieve their goals. Only when you want to get really specific, perhaps for appearing in a bikini competition or on the bodybuilding stage, do you need to do things differently.

The same is true for supplements – women can take just what men take. However, from looking at the supplement industry, and personal experience of producing my own range, it seems that women will only take supplements if they come in pink packets and have feminine names, such as 'Body Tone' or 'Female Sculpt'. Why?

The answer is marketing. We have all been led to believe that women's needs are different, so companies are making a fortune out of creating 'bespoke' female supplements. Again, I ask why? Biologically we are nearly identical. The fact is, apart from hormones, men and women can take the same stuff in the same way.

Have you ever asked what the difference is between male and female supplements? Around 99 per cent of the time it's nothing but the labels. Occasionally, there is a reduction in the amount of each ingredient, presumably because there is a mad idea that women need smaller doses. Women too are offered 'diet' versions of standard products, such as whey protein. The only difference in this case is that it's sold in a pink tub. That's marketing again. So wake up and smell the coffee! You don't need different supplements, you don't need different training plans, and nothing needs to be packaged in pink.

While I'm about it, let's clear up some myths relating to women's training. I often hear them say: 'I don't want to get bulky.' 'I don't want to look masculine.' 'Can I just tone up?' 'I need some exercises to target my abdominal fat.' 'I am on a great new diet where you just drink hot water, lemon juice and cayenne pepper. Is that good for me?'

First, what the hell does 'tone up' mean? Toning up is not a thing; you either train, build muscle and reduce body fat, or you just lose body fat, revealing whatever is underneath. There is no middle ground. You can't do everything except lifting weights in the hope of getting that bikini body you want. You can go on the stepper or cross-trainer for hours, but 'toning up' will elude you, unless you naturally carry more muscle (see Female body shapes, page 19), in which case cardio will reduce your body fat and uncover your natural shape. To put it bluntly, you need to lift weights, do some cardio and eat well to get into shape.

Second, stop worrying about lifting weights. You won't turn into The Hulk, because you lack the testosterone to do so. Not even men go to the gym and suddenly bulk up, however much they would like to think they do. OK, they might go in and get 'pumped' in a particular area they have trained, but that lasts only a short time.

If you have seen a woman who you think looks too bulky, it's because she is happy like that and has probably been working for years to achieve that body. The key thing to understand is that if you train properly, you will have control over what you look like. Everything takes time to change, so remember that before you run scared of the weights.

Sadly, there is a lot of body shaming within our culture, especially among women. I have seen all manner of nasty and negative comments on women's training profiles, and I'm aware of the argument that if you put yourself out there on social media, you deserve whatever comments you get. I don't buy into that, and I don't understand what motivates the viciousness. The problem arises because anyone can voice an opinion anonymously. Just remember this saying, though: 'Opinions are like arseholes. Everybody's got one and thinks everyone else's but their's stinks.'

Oddly, a lot of online nastiness comes from people who are extremely out of shape. The amateur psychologist in me would suggest that they aren't happy with themselves, so they lash out at others. But there's another view that abusers seem keen to perpetuate too. They suggest that being in great shape is disgusting, and that being super-plus size is fine.

If someone is happy being in horrific shape, who am I to say different? All I ask is that they keep their views to themselves. I believe we are each given one body and we should look after it.

WEIGHT OF EXPECTATION

Scales of the weighing variety are not your friends. Well, they are not the kind of friends you want to see every day. I have heard them referred to as the 'naughty step', and while I think that's a little cheesy, it does make a point.

> Scales can destroy or build your confidence within a nanosecond.

Personally, I like to get on them and read big numbers because I want to be heavy and powerful. Some people, though, want the complete opposite; only ever-diminishing numbers will please them. Whatever your goal, scales can play with your head. They can depress, trouble, make you quit, or at the very least think negative thoughts. I recommend you use them in moderation (see page 41).

My wanting to see big numbers is not the whole truth. There is no point seeing 124kg on the dial while looking like a melted wheelie bin. I want to look shredded to the bone when

I see myself in the mirror. (For those of you unfamiliar with the lingo, 'shredded' means healthy but with very low body fat.)

The point I'm trying to make is that we're all aiming for a particular look. All of our goals are appearance based, not weight based.

Unless you are a boxer, you really shouldn't care what the scales say. You could be 5kg heavier than your favoured weight, yet look better than you ever have before. We compare ourselves with others in terms of appearance, not weight, so don't get fixated on the numbers. Do yourself a favour and leave the scales to one side for 95 per cent of this journey. We will use them only occasionally to keep a note of where you are.

For the vast majority of us, weight has nothing to do with what we are trying to achieve. Aesthetics is the only thing that matters, so throw out the scales, or at the very least, hide them away and buy a mirror. (See page 41 for other good ways of tracking your progress.)

YOU ARE NOT MO FARAH

Drive around during the first few weeks of January and you will see everyone up and about, trying to fulfil their new year resolution of getting fit by going out for a run.

Why? Simply because it's easy, and it's what they think they should do. I say wrong, wrong, wrong. Who has ever sat at home and said, **'Do you know what? I love Mo Farah. He is an Olympic legend and I want a body just like his.' The answer is never, except perhaps if you run the 10,000 metres.**

If you have no idea what to do to get fit, running can seem like the simplest and best option. We all know how to run, and running is hard work. It makes us feel like we're doing exercise and thus 'getting into shape'. I've done it myself when I was at school. I used to get all empowered and go for a run to get in shape, but now I know better. You will never get the results you really want by going running.

Let's be honest: it's boring, takes a long time and can hurt your joints. The usual pattern is that someone goes for a couple of runs, then gives up as it's tedious and they don't see their body changing. In my opinion, you are better off doing 20 minutes of bodyweight exercise in your front room than pounding the pavement. I am sure there will be lots of people who will shout me down on this, but it's what I believe. I've got nothing against running to the local park, but when you get there, do some meaningful HIIT training, then run home.

AVOID QUICK FIXES

We live in a world of six-minute abs, meals in 15 seconds and magic pills that can fix everything. I suggest you think of them like payday loans – a quick fix that comes back to haunt you with massive interest.

Similarly, you can go on some mad diet where you drink only a special tea, or wear a corset that squeezes your body into shape, or stop eating major food groups. You will lose weight, but you will put it all back on, and gain it with interest. And this is to say nothing about the side-effects of making yourself ill, run-down or spending most of the time on the loo. It's lunacy, but I actually know people who have done all these things.

Your body is not stupid; it is built for survival. If you starve it, the next time you eat well, it will store more of the food as fat for a rainy day, when you are stupid enough to crash-diet again. Not only that, but it can severely mess up your metabolism and hormones, and, if you are a woman, stop you getting a period.

I recently read a study that suggested almost every woman had tried at least three or four diets in their lifetime. That is a mad statistic, and needs to change. You don't need a diet to change your body. You need sound nutrition. Avoid diets at all costs.

BODY IMAGE

What is the perfect body? To be honest, I have no idea, and if I ever did, my perspective on it has been distorted by looking at others and thinking about what I want to emulate in my own body. I want to be bigger, more ripped, with bigger legs and calves. None of these things have anything to do with making me a better rugby player – they are pure vanity. Nonetheless, they still go through my head on a daily basis. I am never completely happy with what I see in the mirror, but I deal with it by knowing that I am doing everything I can to achieve it while living a happy, balanced life, and making sure my sport of rugby comes first. Don't get me wrong – I don't have body dysmorphia. It's more a desire to keep improving. I think anyone who starts to get results with their body wants to keep pushing to get even more.

Early on in my career I forgot that rugby was all about performance, not about how you looked, and that having a super-low body fat percentage was actually slightly counter-productive. Trying to look like a *Men's Health* cover model should never be a rugby player's aim. Some people, mainly my teammates, would say that with my looks, I am strictly middle pages, or that I have a face for radio, not print.

I had to learn the hard way that I was eating to perform, not eating to look ripped. And I didn't get my nutrition right until I sought expert help. Before then, I'd looked for help online and in magazines, but I was always trying different things. I would start off on one plan, then see something else and move on to that. That's the danger with so much information at our fingertips – we have no way of knowing what is going to work and what we should stick with.

Body image is a huge issue for many people, and it's important to get to grips with it early. You need to be happy in your own skin. That doesn't mean accepting mediocrity. Instead you derive happiness from other things, and don't base it on how you look or how you are perceived. Let's face it, we could all do with improving ourselves and working a bit harder to achieve that, but everything takes time. Make sure you stay focused, keep perspective on where you are and celebrate any small improvements. You have to realise that you are on a journey, and that nobody is ever finished.

You need to have a realistic and attainable idea of what kind of figure you would like. Then, when you reach that goal, you can consider moving to the next step. I have already mentioned genetics as a limiting factor, so my programme can't make you taller, reduce the width of your hips, smooth out knobbly knees, or turn you into an action hero or lingerie model.

Don't be swayed by the 24/7 stream of beautiful people you see on social media. They might have assets you want in your own body, but keep your hopes and wishes real. You don't have to match some (probably Photoshopped) image of perfection. The important thing is to be positive about your own image and the image of those around you.

It was actually my girlfriend who brought this home to me. She said how stupid I was to fall under the spell of social media and its false icons. I had no idea what these people looked like 24/7, how much surgery they'd had, whether they were doped up to the eyeballs with steroids. You, she said, are following false ideals. As usual, she was right. I have followed people on Instagram and got to know their image really well, then innocently walked past them in the street as they looked nothing like their photos. Often, to my embarrassment, they stop to talk to me and I have no idea who they are.

The lesson to learn is that if you to choose to emulate someone, make sure you know for a fact that they eat well, train right and have 100 per cent natural assets. Remember, though, that even the best of them have off days, and that they're not necessarily ripped 24/7.

My last plea is for you to be a good person to others about their body image. I am astounded how spiteful people can be on social media:

> 'Hi, I love that you train and are honest, but you look really manly.' *Tweeted to a number of women I know*

> 'All right chicken legs, don't skip leg day.' *A common theme on most men who train's social media*

If you don't like the way someone does something, or the way someone looks, keep it to yourself. Social media should be a force for good, not a place for nasty people to share their bizarre thoughts.

If you ever find yourself struggling with body image, remember that most people do too. Let's all use this opportunity of following my programme not only to get yourself in shape, but to support those around you in a positive way.

WHAT ARE THEY DOING OVER THERE?

I guarantee that as soon as you tell someone you're starting this programme, they will have an opinion – what you should do, how you should do it, what works or doesn't work. You will find that everyone is an expert. The fact is that fitness, like most other things, can be tackled in a multitude of different ways and there is no short cut to achieving the body you want. Of course, some things will work better than others, but you need to find a programme that you believe in and just do it.

Whenever I post a video online, there are always about 100 comments, and most of them are giving me 'pro tips', such as 'Make sure you squat ass to grass'. That's all well and good, but what happens if I don't have the mobility to do that? I would be putting myself in danger of injury by forcing myself into positions that my body just can't manage.

Another tip might be, 'Do you know what works really well for fat burning? Box jumps.' That's great, but what happens if I have terrible tendonitis in my knees? That exercise is only going to make them worse.

The bottom line is that you need to find a programme that works for you and just get on with it. Give it a chance for six weeks, and if you see no difference, then by all means stop and try something new. Just don't listen to your mate who says, 'You should go swimming, as well as all the other training.' Or the friend who says, 'You need to try intermittent fasting.'

It seems that every person under the sun now has a programme. Fitness is one of the world's fastest-growing industries and everyone is trying to get in on the act. As soon as you say you are reading *Perfect Fit*, someone will suggest you try 'Joe Blogg's 30-day Body Blast', or 'Debbie's Bums and Tums' programme. I implore you to pick just one and do it to the letter, then you can make an informed decision as to what works and what doesn't. Do not become sidetracked.

If you try any outsider's 'tips' while doing my programme, you will hinder your results and not get anything out of it. This is not a mobile phone plan, where you can add helpful bolt-ons. Just stick to what is written, keep it to yourself and give it time to work. Filter the advice you get, and stick to your guns. Ignore stuff that comes from so-called online experts. Most likely it's from a morbidly obese bloke called Dave, who lives in his mum's attic and rarely does more training than waddle to the fridge and back.

As long as you are being safe and working within your limitations, there is no need to add or take away from this plan.

REST DAYS

I want you to train, I want you to eat well and I want you to get results. You will need to train harder than you ever have before, but I have given you an option of two rest days within each normal training week. The reason for this is to give your body time to adapt to the training. I want you to be able to recover so that you can continue to work through the entire programme.

It's not obligatory to take both rest days. Some of you may well want to use one of them to top up certain parts of your training – those areas of personal focus that you want to improve. That is absolutely fine, but you must always take one day off, even if you feel like a million dollars. You cannot train continuously for seven days a week without stressing your body. It's also counter-productive, as it will actually prevent you from getting the results that you want.

More is not better when it comes to training. A lot of the workouts in *Perfect Fit* involve a large number of compound lifts, which use your entire body, not just one specific muscle group. You need to take the rest to allow your muscle fibres to repair and grow stronger.

IF YOU EVER FIND YOURSELF STRUGGLING WITH BODY IMAGE, REMEMBER THAT MOST PEOPLE DO TOO. LET'S ALL USE THIS OPPORTUNITY OF FOLLOWING MY PROGRAMME NOT ONLY TO GET YOURSELF IN SHAPE, BUT TO SUPPORT THOSE AROUND YOU IN A POSITIVE WAY.

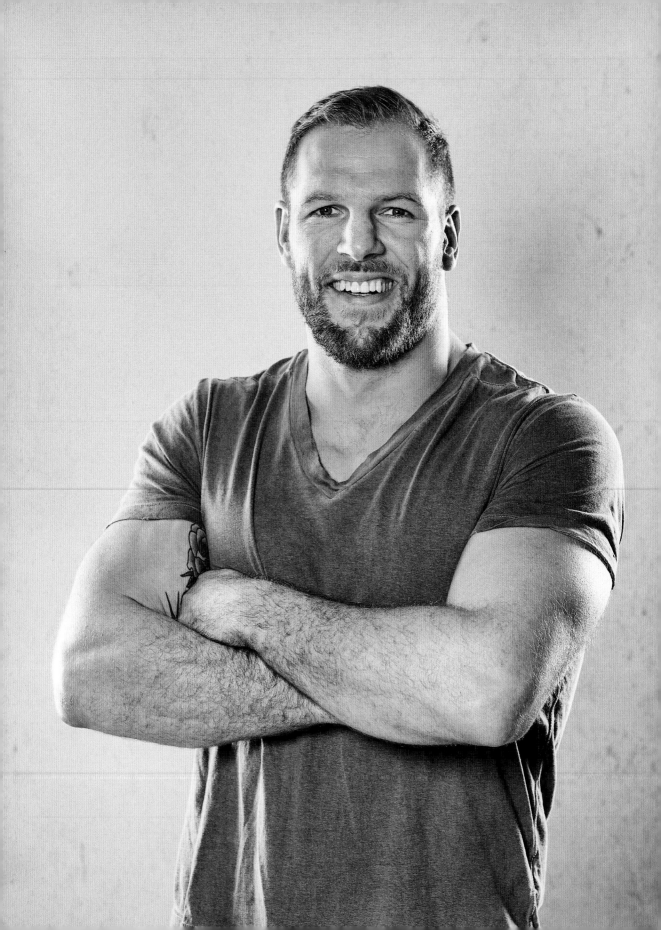

Chapter 2
HOW TO GET THE MOST FROM TRAINING

If you are reading this, let me reassure you that you have made the right decision and bought a book that will deliver results. However, I want you to be aware of the pitfalls that face anyone, from the most experienced trainers to those just starting out. If you set yourself a goal, which in this case is either to lose weight, to lose weight and gain muscle, or just to build muscle, stick absolutely to that one goal. Don't try to become big, fit, strong, lean, fast and powerful all at the same time. It simply won't happen. You need to focus on one thing, and when that ambition has been achieved, you can progress to your next goal, feeling motivated, inspired and confident that you can make it happen.

The only way to get results is to work hard, give up your time and make sacrifices. I have some tips that I think will help you get over the line.

TRAINING TIPS

Find a training partner

Working with a partner who wants to go through this training programme with you will make life so much easier. You can motivate one another when you aren't feeling up to it, you have a ready-made spotter in the gym, and you have a supporter to generally help you train.

Studies have shown that working with a partner, ideally someone who lives under the same roof, increases your chances of getting results and completing the programme. It also helps with staying on point with nutrition and makes mealtimes a breeze, so you aren't eating one thing and they another.

Plan ahead

There is no point buying this book and aiming to follow the programme if you have a stag do, wedding or holiday in the middle of the 12 weeks. I am not saying that you have to map out every aspect of your life in advance, but it's important to earmark a reasonably free span of time when you can commit to the programme. It will be tough enough without having to navigate a social calendar that messes up your nutrition, training and sleep patterns.

Put yourself first

If you want to make changes in your life, especially with your body, you will need to be a little more selfish than usual. **You must put yourself first and say no to anything that will derail this programme. Don't be worried about getting flak from friends and family. If they are true friends, they will understand, and as soon as you start getting results, they will fully support you. You might even find some of them deciding to join in.**

Putting yourself first also means minimising things, such as distractions, lack of sleep and sources of stress that will inhibit your performance. These can massively limit your progress. It's easier said than done to reduce stress, but you have to try because an excess of stress can mess with your hormones and dramatically reduce your performance levels. I have written a whole chapter on the importance of rest and recovery (see page 177), but let me make it clear right here: you need to sleep properly, and four hours a night is just not going to cut it.

While I can't be present in person while you are following this programme, I am still available to offer advice and help. A lot of the most common issues have already been addressed through my social media channels, so if you have a look, you will probably find answers there. If you don't, you can always message me.

Don't be scared of soreness

Soreness is not a bad thing. It shows that you are working hard. However, you must get to grips with the difference between pain and muscle soreness. I suffer terribly from muscle soreness after certain types of workout, but I know that the next day I can push myself through this soreness to perform another session. Chapter 5 deals with recovery and mobility and offers tips for reducing soreness. The idea of the 12-week programme is to push you into a phase of over-reaching, not over-training. This means pushing your body so it creates changes in metabolism and muscle tissue. **You need to embrace the fact that working hard means some discomfort, a certain amount of pain and often being completely out of breath. In all likelihood, you will also be thinking, 'What the hell am I doing here?'**

Choose the right weight

When you come to lift weights in this programme, make sure you choose the right one. I can't suggest what will work for you as I don't know you personally. What I do know is that if you want your body to change, you need to challenge it and put your muscles under tension. Many people lift too light, which means they won't get the results they should. Women, I'm sorry to say, are huge culprits of this. I walk into a gym and see a woman doing set after set using the 4kg dumbbells. I then see her leave the gym with a suitcase-sized handbag that probably weighs more like 12kg.

Ladies, you need to push yourselves, lift heavier and stop faffing around. Do not be afraid of discomfort – it's a good thing.

There is, of course, the gym-goer who does exactly the opposite and lifts way too heavy. This means that their technique is terrible, their range of movement is appalling and they fail to finish the workout. The sets and reps in this programme are designed to get the best out of you, so I urge you to choose a weight that challenges you and makes the last three reps of every set a struggle. Whether you need to increase your lift or drop it down, do it. Put your ego on hold for the greater good of getting into sick-ass shape.

HOW TO PREPARE FOR TRAINING

A lot depends on whether you are training in the morning, the afternoon, or a couple of times during the day. My expectations of what you should do are outlined in Chapter 3 at the beginning of both the 8-week and 12-week programmes. In either case, there are a number of useful things you can do before starting a training session. These are outlined below and will help you to get the best out of your workouts.

Keep hydrated

I always start my day with a focus on hydration. Every morning before I leave for training I drink 1.5–2 litres of water mixed with an electrolyte supplement. The idea is to provide the body with the salts and minerals that have been lost while sleeping. I am always very dehydrated in the mornings, and if I don't address this, I feel rubbish and underperform. You don't have to drink as much as I do, but try to have at least 500ml of water with or without an electrolyte tablet or powder.

In programmes like those in this book, you are asked to work very hard, so hydration cannot ever be taken for granted. You need to nail this, and one way is to get yourself a good water bottle and monitor how many times you drain and refill it.

Eat well

Effective training goes hand in hand with good nutrition, and comprehensive information on this subject is given in Chapter 6. Nutrition is definitely *not* an area where 'one size fits all': some of you have trained before, others haven't; some of you need to lose weight, while others are skinny and find it hard to put on size. Your needs are individual, so Chapter 6 gives you the tools to work out your own bespoke nutrition plan, specifying calories, number of meals and much more. Use this in conjunction with the delicious recipes in Chapter 7 and you will be certain of success.

Consider taking a pre-trainer supplement

Tough workout sessions take lots of energy, and using a pre-trainer supplement can really give you a boost to get you through, especially if you have to get up early and train before work. Using supplements is also something that you can try as training gets more intense. However, there is no obligation to do so. You might decide that supplements are a step too far.

If you do decide to try a pre-trainer, make sure it's Informed Sport Tested so you can be sure it's high quality. There is detailed information about how to choose an appropriate one on page 214.

If you don't want to fork out money on supplements, you can make your own at home. It won't be quite as good, but it will get the job done.

The simplest form of pre-trainer is a double shot of espresso, which does the trick if you are just aiming to burn fat. Alternatively, blend a double shot of espresso with a teaspoonful of coconut oil or MCT oil. The caffeine will wake you up and boost your concentration, while the oil will give you energy.

You could also try using caffeine chewing gum just before training or playing. I use it a lot.

You can also legitimately consume energy drinks, such as Lucozade and Powerade, during workouts, but I would avoid them at all other times as they contain a lot of empty calories in the form of sugar.

Warm up

Before you go into any session, you need to spend some time warming up properly. This will help you to avoid injuries and set you up to hit the ground running. You don't want to ease into your workout, you want to use the limited time you have to work to the max.

A warm-up routine is given with the training plans (see page 45).

If you have mobility issues, I recommend you a read book by Dr. Kelly Starrett called *Becoming a Supple Leopard*. It provides solutions to most common problems, such as tight hamstrings and stiff shoulders, but it also changed the way I approach my training and has made a big difference to any mobility issues I am having. Also check out the recovery chapter of this book (see page 177), where there are a few simple ways to work on your mobility. Little moves, such as foam rolling or banded stretching, before you go into the actual warm-up are really helpful.

I know it sounds like yet more work, but you will thank me when you get through the training programme unscathed and are able to progress even further.

WHEN SHOULD I TRAIN?

To put it bluntly, it's not important what time of day you train. I happen to hate training in the morning. I much prefer late afternoon or evening because I have much more energy than at other times of day. It's the same for other people too. Just look at the legendary boxer Floyd Mayweather: he would only ever train late at night.

I have mentioned before about finding a programme that can be personalised to fit around your lifestyle, but here are a few things to bear in mind. If you are aiming only to lose weight, training fasted (on an empty stomach) in the morning can be useful. There is no conclusive evidence that this will hugely affect your weight loss, but the idea behind it is that if you haven't eaten for at least eight hours, you will use up your body's stores of carbohydrate and then start using your body fat as fuel. It makes sense, so why wouldn't it work?

The one thing that has been proven is that training fasted will boost your metabolism, which will carry on through the day and help you to burn up calories.

> A word of warning: under no circumstances should you ever train fasted for the resistance sessions in the plan, and especially not for the very tough lifting workouts in the full 12-week programme.

What is important is to train when you can, making sure you allocate enough time to complete the sessions properly and in depth.

YOU NEED TO FOCUS ON ONE THING, AND WHEN THAT AMBITION HAS BEEN ACHIEVED, YOU CAN PROGRESS TO YOUR NEXT GOAL FEELING MOTIVATED, INSPIRED AND CONFIDENT.

TYPES OF TRAINING USED IN *PERFECT FIT*

Bodyweight training

(also known as callisthenics) is a really useful tool to help you achieve your fitness goals. It is for everyone, not just beginners, but if you have never trained before, this is a great place to start your fitness journey. You can't really go wrong with bodyweight work. Some of the strongest, most in-shape people I know started with bodyweight work, and still use it all the time in their programmes. Bodyweight training also reduces the risk of injury and allows you to develop and build a good foundation.

Only once you have cracked this can you progress to lifting weights. The first eight weeks is set up so you can get used to training and use the best tool at your disposal, which is your bodyweight. The other bonus of bodyweight work is that you can do it anywhere, so it is great at home, on holiday and staying fit on the go. There is no need for a gym. I spend a lot of my time doing bodyweight work on a daily basis.

German volume training

(aka Ten-set volume method) is used only in the 12-week plan. It has been around for a long time and is very popular with both professional and amateur weightlifters and bodybuilders. They often use this type of programme in their off-seasons to pack on volume (size).

In the past, when I have been recovering from injury or surgery and needed to build muscles during the rehab period, I always employed this type of training. On the last occasion, I spent six weeks doing this work non-stop and, as a result, greatly reduced my rehab time. I also put on a large amount of muscle very quickly, far faster than with anything else I have done. The programme works because it exposes muscle fibres to extraordinary stress. Basically, an exercise targeting a particular muscle is performed for 10 sets and causes the cells to hypertrophy (thicken or increase in size).

German volume training works in a couple of ways: 10 sets of 10 reps, or 10 sets of 6–8 reps.

HIIT (High-Intensity Interval Training)

aims to burn fat while retaining muscle. As an added bonus, it continues to burn fat for many hours after you have finished training.

HIIT is a form of cardio work that involves a series of very intense exercises requiring 90 per cent or more of maximum heart rate. It includes things such as running on the spot and burpees followed by a series of low-intensity exercises, such as walking recovery or rest. The split would be 20–40 seconds of intense work, and 45–90 seconds of rest, so the pattern is high intensity, low intensity.

For most people, short sessions of HIIT (say, 20 minutes) are more likely to help preserve lean muscle tissue than long spurts of cardio. Also, a 20-minute session is easier to knuckle down to than spending hours in the gym going through the monotony of straight-up cardio training.

HIIT not only helps to burn fat, it also gets you really fit. It's something I use very often to prepare for the rigours of a rugby game.

At the time of writing, bodyweight training is hugely in fashion, and something that people are favouring over weights. Remember, it's not all about what you can squat or bench.

LISS (Low-Intensity Steady-State cardio)

is used for optional extra sessions on days off or for top-ups. It is the classic type of cardio training that you see most people doing in the gym – sustained, low-intensity work that often takes around 30–60 minutes to complete. When performing LISS, you can wear a heart-rate monitor to make sure you are keeping your levels in the optimum zone, which for most people is 120–150 beats per minute (bpm). If you don't have a monitor, the optimum zone is when you are working neither too hard nor too little. This means your oxygen level is such that you can just about hold a conversation while working out.

A little tip on cardio training: if you have to do it, and you are doing it along with weight training, I suggest you do it after you have lifted your weights. You don't want to be tired out for your lifting session, as that is the most important workout of the day. Being tired can affect form and dramatically diminish the intensity of the session. It's also important to note that lifting weights in itself creates a fat-burning effect in the body, which will be multiplied by doing cardio after or during a separate session that day.

Resistance training

must be done using weight, and is the key to getting bigger and building muscle. The idea behind resistance training is to put force through your muscle fibres to cause micro tears, which then heal with new tissue, thus creating muscle development. You need to lift the right amount of weight to cause these changes to happen. Resistance is the most classic form of training and something that gym-goers will be familiar with. The sessions in this programme are based around time-under-tension work and load, which is all about building muscle.

You will see in the training guide that for every workout and week, I suggest the correct tempo at which you should be lifting weights. It's really important to follow this because the amount of time your muscles are under tension with the correct load, the more muscle fibres become damaged and the more likely it is you are going to promote growth of new muscle tissue.

We will be looking to do more repetitions, 10 reps or more, in order to build size, as opposed to smaller rep counts with heavier weights, which are designed to develop strength.

You will of course see strength gains throughout this programme as a matter of course. The positives of resistance training vastly outweigh the negatives.

Building lean muscle mass raises your base metabolic rate because your body burns more calories in order to support that higher mass. Similar to HIIT cardio (see page 35), resistance training can burn calories for up to 48 hours post-workout, as well as repairing and building new muscle tissue.

Weighted vs bodyweight work

Options are sometimes given for doing weighted or bodyweight versions of certain exercises. The idea is to do whatever you feel capable of. For example, you might be able to do only bodyweight exercises, but as you go through the programme, you should aim to start adding some weight, or to start doing the weighted versions of those exercises. If you find the bodyweight work too easy, you can also look to weight the first couple of sets of, say, chin-ups, and as you get tired, you can drop back down to bodyweight only.

You need to check your ego at the door. Yes, lads – I'm speaking to you. If you have ever looked at The Rock or any male fitness icon and wondered how much he benches, or how much he squats, you are a prime candidate for this word of warning. Anyone can lift a heavy weight really badly, and anyone can do a half-rep, or try to shift weights really quickly. Doing it properly is what you should be looking for.

FORM AND TECHNIQUE

Both German volume training and resistance training require you to lift weights, but the form in which you lift is far more important than the amount you lift. By 'form', I am referring to your technique and how you look whilst lifting. Type 'terrible deadlift technique' into YouTube and you will see any number of idiots manhandling large amounts of weight any way they can. This not only looks crazy, but could potentially cause significant injury.

> The training plans in this book are about pushing yourself to acquire perfect technique and form. Women often underlift, while men often overlift, so please, all of you, remember we are trying to build something here that will take time.

In Chapter 4 you will find a step-by-step description of every single exercise, along with really clear photographs of what you should look like while doing it. If this isn't enough, go online and find the correct technique in action, making sure you watch videos only from reputable trainers or well-established websites. As always, do your due diligence on the information and people you are following. Please don't end up being that person who features on a social media page like Gym Fails, using the leg extension as a neck trainer, or who appears to be having some kind of fit while trying to do a lat pull down.

I have worked with a lot people and heard many excuses about why they lift poorly. If only they would follow this simple rule: if you can't squat properly, don't squat with a weight. Go back a stage or two and learn how to do a really good bodyweight squat. Similarly, if you

can't do a press-up but can bench press, you aren't clever or cool, you are a muppet. Take that back a stage or two as well, and learn to perform a press-up properly with control before progressing to a bench press.

Young lads are the worst offenders. They all want to be the big dogs in the gym, claiming they can squat this and bench that. I took a group of 16-year-olds through a workout recently and all they wanted to know was how to lift weights. I started a couple of them off with barbell squats, and it was horrific viewing. As a result, I took them back to bodyweight squats, and most of them couldn't do that well either. They were all trying to run before they could walk. My message to them, as it is to you, is that lifting weights properly is a skill. You need to start with the basics. I often go righ back to basics when I start a new rugby season.

I strip off all the weight on the bar and go back to perfect form and range of motion. I could 'squat' 300kg by taking the bar off, dropping down a couple of inches, then driving back up. I'd be able to tell everyone I could do it, but what would be the point? The fact of the matter is that it's not really a squat. Far better would be to go down to 100kg, squatting as low as I can while maintaining excellent form and the full range of movement. If I have five reps to do and I can do all five perfectly, I stay on 100kg or I slightly increase the weight for the next set. It all depends on how easy I found it. If I have five reps to do and I can do only one that looks great, I drop the weight down to 80kg and I go again until I can do the five reps properly.

> Remember, we are training for life, not just for 8 or 12 weeks. Give yourself time to develop your form and get the most out of this book.

TRAINING TERMINOLOGY

Like any specialist subject, fitness has its own jargon and this can be a little off-putting to beginners. Don't be alarmed – the following guide (in alphabetical order) will make everything clear.

Athletic position

this is the way you should stand at the beginning of an exercise. The basic form is feet shoulder width apart, knees slightly bent, abdominal muscles engaged, shoulders set. The stance may vary a little, depending on what you are being asked to do, but these are the key points always to think about. You should feel ready for action.

Bias

a focus more on one side than the other.

Concentric

the raising phase of any weightlifting exercise.

DOMS

Delayed Onset Muscle Soreness, the after-effect of training hard.

Drive

to concentrically move the weight back up in a dynamic manner.

Dynamic

energetic and fast.

Eccentric

the lowering phase of any weightlifting exercise.

Explode

to move as powerfully as you can.

Floss

to make a small backward and forward motion in a muscle to gradually stretch it out and increase its range.

Form

the way in which you perform each exercise.

Full body

a session or exercise focused on training the entire body.

Half-rep

half the possible range of movement that can be done in an exercise.

ITB

iliotibial band, also known as Maissiat's band or IT band, is a thick strip of connective tissue in the thigh that helps with flexion and extension of the knee.

Loading phase

the initial 5–10 days when you begin taking a supplement, e.g. creatine, in order to build up the levels of it in the body. The loading phase is followed by a maintenance phase, when a lower dosage is taken.

Lower body exercise

a session focused solely on developing the lower body from the hips down.

Reps

repetitions; the number of times a specific exercise is repeated.

Rest

the time taken to recover after working out, or the down time between sets.

Set

a full block of exercises, e.g. 1a.

Snap

to move briskly from one position to another.

Stand-alone exercise

an exercise performed for a specified number of sets before you move on to the next.

Superset

a set of two exercises (a, b) performed straight after one another before resting, then repeating in exactly the same way. There is occasionally a slight variation on this, where you do set A, then go on to B and rest, then start again.

Tempo

the speed at which weights are lifted. The raising phase is known as 'concentric', and the lowering phase as 'eccentric'. The tempo is often written with three numbers, e.g. 3.1.3. This means 3 seconds to lower, 1 second pause, 3 seconds to raise again.

Tense

to engage a muscle group, as in 'tense your glutes'.

Traps

trapezius muscles: two large muscles in the back that extend vertically from the base of the skull to the shoulder blades. They are essential for rotation and support.

Tri-set

a set of three exercises (a, b, c) performed in that order before resting, and then repeated in exactly the same way. Or you rest after A, then onto B, rest after B and then onto C. Rest and then start again. Both variations are used in this book.

Upper body exercise

a session focused solely on developing the upper body from the hips up.

HOW TO TRACK YOUR RESULTS

It is hugely important to track your results, and this must begin on the very first day of training. You need to take some baseline readings of yourself – height, weight, measurements, BMR and TDEE (see page 191) – as starting points from which to track your progress. Thereafter it's important to continue tracking consistently, using the same methods every time. Not doing so will derail your progress and have a big effect on you mentally. Make sure you follow the rules for each of the tracking methods outlined below.

FOCUS ON WHAT
YOU CAN CONTROL,
WHICH IS YOURSELF.
IF YOU HAVE ANY
DOUBTS, ASK YOURSELF
IF YOU ARE HONESTLY
DOING EVERYTHING
YOU POSSIBLY CAN
TO GET INTO SHAPE.

Take photos

In my opinion, photos are probably the best way of tracking yourself, as they clearly show how you change over time, but please note the following rules.

You are not trying to take a perfect selfie, but how you take the photos is super-important. Do ensure you take them in the same location, ideally wearing the same clothes and in the same conditions. This means the same time of day, same lighting and same aspect, if possible. These things will make a big difference to how you look because your appearance before meals, for example, is different from after meals, and your level of hydration will also affect the way you look.

I believe it's best to take photos in your pants or underwear in the morning, just after you have woken up, and before breakfast. Remember what lights, if any, you have on, and exactly where you are standing.

In order to see a clear indication of the progress you are making, I suggest that you take photos every two weeks. Don't take a photo every day as the changes will be very difficult to detect and you will get disheartened.

Please feel free to share your photos with us at *Perfect Fit*: we love to see how you are getting on. Simply tweet @jameshaskell, tag us on Instagram @jamehask, or email jhfitnessblog@gmail.com.

Weigh yourself

As with all tracking methods, do ensure you weigh yourself at the same time of the day, wearing the same clothes and always using the same set of scales. If you chop and change scales, you will see discrepancies that might set you back.

Whatever you do, don't weigh yourself every day – it will mess with your head. Weight is so easily affected by variables, such as your level of hydration and when you last ate, that it's not the most helpful marker of progress. It's certainly not worth obsessing over.

I prefer photos as the camera never lies, whereas the scales very often provide a misleading result. Do not become hung up on weight! We are striving for personal aesthetic perfection, so if you look and feel amazing, it really doesn't matter if you are heavier than you want.

It must be said – women are generally more likely than men to become obsessed with weight. It's not healthy, and worrying about what the scales say is not going to bring you the results you want, or the happiness and fulfilment you are looking for. Some people seem to regard controlling their weight as gaining control over their life. That thinking just doesn't stack up. Life is far too unpredictable to control, and it's an illusion to think that you can impose control on it through your body and weight. Do not seek control in this way; it only leads down a much darker path. Instead, see weight as a guide, but consider how you feel and look as far more important.

Having said this, I know weight obsession is not exclusive to women. I have seen many men, particularly those in professional sport, fall into the same trap. Not a day goes by without some players worrying if they have gained or lost weight. It's not healthy, and some teams have stopped tracking it pre-match because it can have an adverse phychological effect to find that you are a few kilos lighter than you thought. You start thinking, 'Does this make me weak or less powerful?' You then go into the game distracted and anxious, when you should be filled with confidence.

Take your measurements

Another useful way to track your progress is to take your measurements every two weeks and record them. It's best to photocopy this and to place it alongside your progression photos where you can easily see them. The fridge door is a good place, as every time you open it to put something into your body, the display will be a positive reminder of how you are getting on and why it's important to stay on track.

To take your measurements, use a fabric tape measure, the kind used by tailors. Also, decide in advance whether you are going to record things in centimetres or inches. Remember, consistency is essential.

The areas you should look to keep track of are as follows:

> » **Thighs/quad muscles –** measure at the widest point
> » **Chest –** measure around the widest point
> » **Waist –** measure around the middle at the narrowest point
> » **Arms/biceps –** measure the widest part while flexing the muscle
> » **Calf –** measure the widest part

Measure your body fat

We want this training programme to be a really positive and fun process, so it is not essential to track your body fat – you will see it quite clearly in the photos you take. However, if you must do it, make sure you are consistent in the method you use. We don't want you being derailed by some anomalous results.

There are several ways of measuring body fat, so make sure you stick to the same method throughout your training.

>> **Bod pod** – a small machine that calculates body density by measuring the air displaced when someone sits inside it. There are specialist places you can visit to have this done.

>> **Callipers** – a simple measuring device, often used by nutritionists, but also available in gyms. The technique is to use the fingers to pinch a fold of skin at various sites on the body, e.g. chest, arms, abs and thighs, then use callipers to measure it.

>> **DEXA scan** – a form of X-ray that uses low-energy beams to measure fat mass. It gives very accurate results and is usually done at a hospital or clinic, but is sometimes available from mobile units.

>> **Electronic reader** – a type of scale that incorporates electrodes on which you stand. In my experience, you can get up to a 10 per cent difference between electronic readers (they always have me as morbidly obese).

Don't make comparisons

Never compare your progress to another person's. I feel really strongly about this. We've all done it and it never goes well.

Everyone makes progress at different rates, so do not be discouraged by what you see others doing or achieving. Focus on what you can control, which is yourself. If you have any doubts, ask yourself if you are honestly doing everything you possibly can to get into shape. This is far more constructive than looking over your shoulder at others.

My father taught me that you can lie to everyone else but you can't lie to yourself. So before you start panicking and think of throwing in the towel because others are getting results faster than you, take a good, hard look at yourself and ask, 'Could I do better?' In 99 per cent of cases, I suspect the answer will be yes. It certainly is when I ask myself. So go at it with renewed intensity and focus on your own results, not others'.

Chapter 3
THE TRAINING PLANS

Perfect Fit is designed to be used by everyone, regardless of size, weight or level of fitness. That's why this chapter starts with a simple 8-week training plan that you don't need a gym for. You can try it and learn that you can get great results without having to pay for gym membership. It's also ideal for those who have never really trained before.

As far as I'm concerned, you can argue till the cows come home that you don't have time to work out, but I guarantee that if I sat down with you, we could always find time for a workout.

> One thing I learnt early on in my fitness and rugby career was never to set goals that I wouldn't fulfil. It's just demoralising. For example, telling yourself that you will train every day for an hour is silly, especially if you have never trained before. You will never do it. Far better is to say, 'I am going to train for 10 minutes on one day a week' and progress from there. You will quickly see you have more time than you think – we all do – and 10 minutes once a week, twice a week, then four times a week is very possible.

If you are new to training or are in dire need of shifting some weight, the 8-week plan is the best place to start. The first four weeks focus on bodyweight training, which requires no equipment.

The second four weeks introduces you to basic gym stuff, but you can stick with the bodyweight training if you want to. The idea is that you can move up to the next level as and when you feel ready.

If you wish to do the full 12-week plan, you will definitely need access to a gym. If you don't want to go that far, you can simply repeat the 8-week plan, or even just the first four weeks of it, as many times as you like. You will still burn fat, lose weight and start to develop muscles and definition.

If you do decide to repeat all or part of the 8-week plan, all you have to do is increase the time for each exercise. This can be done in 5-second increments while slightly reducing the rest time according to how tired you are. That's the beauty of this training programme: even if you do the 12-week plan, you can change things to suit yourself, perhaps going back to the 8-week plan while you're on holiday, or cherry-picking certain workouts.

The beginner's plan will get you into great shape as long as you eat well with it. The nutrition chapter (see page 189) gives a detailed explanation of how to do that, but the principles are very simple. If you want to lose weight and improve definition, you eat carbohydrates only on your training days post workout. If you want to build muscle, you eat carbs every day. In both cases, you will only see the benefit of eating in these ways if you actually train.

Carbs are not for everyone all the time. Weight-losers need to earn them by cashing in a tough training session.

By all means skip ahead to page 189 and read the nutrition chapter if you want, but at this stage there is no need to get deeply involved in that information. I suggest you focus just on pages 190–193 as these will help you to eat well for your chosen goal.

GET READY

As discussed in Chapter 2, it's essential to warm up before a training session, and to recover properly afterwards. See the routine described opposite and on page 184, and be sure to follow them to get the best results from training and to avoid injury.

WARM-UP ROUTINE

The following warm-up can be used with both training plans. I recommend doing it before any session. The idea is to warm up your core temperature and get your heart beating faster. This is especially important when doing high-impact interval training (HIIT), as you don't want to go into that stiff and cold.

Even if you're only lifting weights in a session, I still recommend doing something to get you moving and increase your heart rate. Say you have five sets of squats, you need to do 2–4 warm-up ones early on to build up to your start weight. This will be the same for most exercises, and, more often than not, is applicable to the very first lift of the day. You can then go straight into the first set of exercises following this, but take the time you need to get things right.

To give you an exact example of how this works, you do 2–4 warm-up sets for your first lift, which might be a back squat. Then, when you move on to the deadlift, you might need only one or two warm-up sets to get you going. That's why it's really important to keep a log of your starting and finishing weights for each session. Also, don't be timid. Some people are scared to lift heavy in case they injure themselves, so they always lift the same. Others go heavy too quickly and burn out. Your body needs constant change to grow, so increase gradually – perhaps by a couple of kilos per session if you feel you can. Don't be afraid to push yourself.

The overall message I want to leave you with is that warm-ups should be dynamic – they should contain movement that engages the muscles you are about to train. They should prepare you for whatever session you're doing.

You will be focusing on this warm-up for roughly 10 minutes, or until you feel ready to start. I suggest doing each exercise for 30–60 seconds, and doing a couple of rounds of each exercise overall, to take up the full 10 minutes. However, you can take as little or as much time as you want to get moving.

If you are using this warm-up for the full 12-week programme, you could also jump on a piece of cardio equipment, such as a Wattbike or treadmill, and perform 4–6 minutes of gradual work before going into the mobility work below, which should be completed in the order listed. You want to come out of the warm-up with your heart rate raised and your body ready to participate fully in the session. You can spend longer warming up if you feel you need longer to reach that point. Full descriptions of each exercise can be found in Chapter 4.

>> **Back roll-outs** perform for 1 minute, making sure you feel fully loose.
>> **Russian twists** do 6–10 on each side, trying to go further each time, and feel your lower back loosen out.
>> **Running on the spot high knees** perform for 30 seconds.
>> **Running on the spot butt kicks** perform for 30 seconds.
>> **Star jumps** perform dynamically, i.e. fast, for 30 seconds.
>> **Hamstring walkout** perform 6 full reps.
>> **Lunge drills** do four types of lunge: forward, reverse, lateral and curtsey. Perform 3 complete rounds of each one.
>> **Press-ups** perform 10, but change your hand position after every second one. This means you start in the normal position, do two press-ups, then take your hands slightly wider for the next two, then wider again, then narrower and narrower until you're back in the start position. You can also do press-ups with your hands unevenly spaced.

8-WEEK TRAINING PLAN FOR BEGINNERS

The first four weeks of the programme alternate between one day of HIIT training and one day of resistance training.

You are training once a day, and have been given two days off per week. To get the most out of the programme you need to be training 4–5 times a week. If you do that, you will see the amazing results you are after.

You can, however, use one of those days off to perform an extra session if you want. It all depends on how you feel and how your body is reacting. If you go for it, simply repeat one of the HIIT sessions from your training plan, or choose a LISS session (see page 174), or repeat any resistance session from the week you are currently engaged in.

PLEASE NOTE
Do not do the same training session two days in a row.
You must take one of the days off for complete rest.

You will mostly be working for 20 seconds flat out within the HIIT sessions, with a rest period of 45–60 seconds. The idea behind this spectrum of rest is to make sure that everyone, regardless of fitness level, will be able to get some benefit from these sessions. For example, if I were doing the HIIT sessions, I would be looking to take a maximum of

45 seconds rest. This means that by the end of the workout I would be shattered. You the reader are not tied to that: you can choose exactly how hard to push yourself, and adapt proceedings to your particular fitness level. If you can't complete the workout taking 60 seconds rest between sets, you can rest for 90 seconds instead. However, this is for those who are extremely unfit or who are just returning to training.

The idea is for you to work as hard as you can, take enough rest to feel refreshed, then to repeat the next rep with the same intensity as the first. Obviously, as you get towards the middle and end of the session, you will see a drop in your intensity level, but that's supposed to happen if you're working properly.

For the resistance sessions you will see that the rest period is 60–80 seconds. Again, this is to help those of mixed ability complete the sessions and get the most out of them. Make sure you are strict about getting your rest.

In some sessions you have a choice of exercises, which are separated by slash marks. These are simply options: there is no such thing as best. Those highlighted in grey are options for people who might not want to develop that particular area of their body, or for reasons of strength and current ability might need a pared-down version of it. Or because you have access to limited equipment so need clever alternatives to do instead. For example, normal press-ups can be done instead of kneeling press-ups, but the choice is entirely yours, and you might not choose to make any substitutions.

The training plan is split into weeks, which are subdivided into 1–5 sessions. While you are free to rearrange them around your work and personal schedule, I suggest you keep to things the way they are set out so that you don't inadvertently miss a session, fail to get the best results, or overtrain a certain body part. You must not skip sessions because you don't like them or find them too hard. You need to complete the workouts, so if you are struggling, take a few steps back and do the most basic form of the exercise.

SUMMARY OF THE 8-WEEK PLAN

Here is an overview of how the 8 weeks look in term of intensity:

Weeks 1 & 2 »	Low to medium intensity
Weeks 3–6 »	Medium intensity
Weeks 7 & 8 »	Medium to high intensity

FOCUS ON WHAT YOU CAN CONTROL, WHICH IS YOURSELF

ALWAYS READ THE INSTRUCTIONS

As the training plan progresses, there are little changes at the start of each week and section. Do not assume that you know what the week holds, or how you are going to be training. Make sure you always read the text at the start of the week. If there is no new information there, it's business as usual and the week is the same as the previous one.

Please refer to the photos and descriptions of the exercises in Chapter 4 to make sure you are doing things correctly.

» **Remember to do a warm-up routine** before every workout session (see page 45).

» **Days off** – you have the option to fully rest, but if you prefer, you can do a LISS session (see page 174), or perform another HIIT or resistance session, depending on what your goal is, how you feel and the results you want to get. Do remember, though, that recovery is very important. Please refer to the recovery and mobility advice in Chapter 5 (see page 177), where various options – ice baths, foam rolling, compression garments and so forth – are discussed.

» **Make sure you check** whenever you are required to do standalone exercises or supersets at the start of every session.

8-WEEK TRAINING PLAN WEEK 1

SESSION 1 HIIT, STAND-ALONE EXERCISES

1 Running on the spot »
20 seconds work, 45–60 seconds rest, 8 sets.

2 Star jumps »
20 seconds work, 45–60 seconds rest, 8 sets.

3 Mountain climbers »
20 seconds work, 45–60 seconds rest, 8 sets.

SESSION 2 RESISTANCE, UPPER BODY, STAND-ALONE EXERCISES, TEMPO 3.1.3

1 Press-ups/Kneeling press-ups/ Wall press-ups »
10 reps, 60–80 seconds rest, 3 sets.

2 Bodyweight squats »
10 reps, 60–80 seconds rest, 3 sets.

3 Walking lunges/Forward lunges »
10 reps (5 each side), 60–80 seconds rest, 3 sets.

DAY OFF

SESSION 3 HIIT, STAND-ALONE EXERCISES

1 Boxing while running on the spot »
20 seconds work, 45–60 seconds rest, 8 sets.

2 Side-to-side hops »
20 seconds work, 45–60 seconds rest, 8 sets.

3 Bodyweight slams »
20 seconds work, 45–60 seconds rest, 8 sets.

SESSION 4 RESISTANCE, FULL BODY, STAND-ALONE EXERCISES, TEMPO 3.1.3

1 Step-ups »
10 reps (5 each side), 60–80 seconds rest, 3 sets.

2 Wide hand placement press-ups/ Kneeling wide hand press-ups/Wide hand placement wall press-ups »
10 reps, 60–80 seconds rest, 3 sets.

3 Front plank »
20–30 seconds hold, 60–80 seconds rest, 4 sets.

SESSION 5 HIIT, STAND-ALONE EXERCISES

1 Squat jumps »
20 seconds work, 45–60 seconds rest, 8 sets.

2 Burpees/Down and ups »
20 seconds work, 45–60 seconds rest, 8 sets.

3 Side-lying opens »
20 seconds work, 45–60 seconds rest, 8 sets.

DAY OFF

8-WEEK TRAINING PLAN WEEK 2

SESSION 1 HIIT, STAND-ALONE EXERCISES

1 Running on the spot »
20 seconds work, 45–60 seconds rest, 8 sets.

2 Speed walk-out press-up »
20 seconds work, 45–60 seconds rest, 8 sets.

3 Rotational chops »
20 seconds work, 45–60 seconds rest, 8 sets.

SESSION 2 RESISTANCE, FULL BODY, STAND-ALONE EXERCISES

1 Incline press-ups/Kneeling press-ups/Wall press-ups »
10 reps, 60–80 seconds rest, 3 sets.

2 Bodyweight squats »
10 reps, 60–80 seconds rest, 3 sets.

3 Bodyweight bench dips (use a bench, box or chair) »
10 reps, 60–80 seconds rest, 3 sets.

4 Walking lunges/Forward lunges »
10 reps, 60–80 seconds rest, 3 sets.

DAY OFF

SESSION 3 HIIT, STAND-ALONE EXERCISES

1 Side-to-side hops »
20 seconds work, 45–60 seconds rest, 8 sets.

2 Mountain climber/Hop forwards and backwards on the spot »
20 seconds work, 45–60 seconds rest, 8 sets.

3 Skier swing »
20 seconds work, 45–60 seconds rest, 8 sets.

SESSION 4 RESISTANCE, STAND-ALONE EXERCISES, TEMPO 3.1.3

1 Step-up (use a box, chair or bench) »
10 reps (5 each side), 60–80 seconds rest, 3 sets.

2 Narrow hand placement press-up/Kneeling narrow hand placement press-up/Narrow hand placement wall press-ups »
10 reps, 60–80 seconds rest, 3 sets.

3 Sumo squat »
10 reps, 60–80 seconds rest, 3 sets.

4 Glute bridge »
10 reps, 60–80 seconds rest, 3 sets.

SESSION 5 HIIT, STAND-ALONE EXERCISES

1 Broad jump to backward hop »
20 seconds work, 45–60 seconds, 8 sets.

2 Front plank/Front plank with hand tap »
20 seconds work, 45–60 seconds, 8 sets.

3 Star jump »
20 seconds work, 45–60 seconds, 8 sets.

DAY OFF

8-WEEK TRAINING PLAN WEEK 3

SESSION 1 HIIT, STAND-ALONE EXERCISES

1 Running on the spot »
20 seconds work, 45–60 seconds rest, 8 sets.

2 Star jump »
20 seconds work, 45–60 seconds rest, 8 sets.

3 Mountain climber »
20 seconds work, 45–60 seconds rest, 8 sets.

SESSION 2 RESISTANCE, UPPER BODY, STAND-ALONE EXERCISES, TEMPO 3.1.3

1 Press-up/Kneeling press-up/ Wall press-up »
10 reps, 60–80 seconds rest, 3 sets.

2 Bodyweight squat »
10 reps, 60–80 seconds rest, 3 sets.

3 Bodyweight slam »
10 reps (5 each side), 60–80 seconds rest, 3 sets.

DAY OFF

SESSION 3 HIIT, STAND-ALONE EXERCISES

1 Boxing while running on the spot »
20 seconds work, 45–60 seconds rest, 8 sets.

2 Side-to-side hops »
20 seconds work, 45–60 seconds rest, 8 sets.

3 Bodyweight slam »
20 seconds work, 45–60 seconds rest, 8 sets.

SESSION 4 RESISTANCE, FULL BODY, STAND-ALONE EXERCISES, TEMPO 3.1.3

1 Step-up (use a box, chair or bench) »
10 reps (5 each side), 60–80 seconds rest, 3 sets.

2 Wide press-up/Kneeling wide press-up/Wide wall press-up »
10 reps, 60–80 seconds rest, 3 sets.

3 Front plank »
20–30 seconds hold, 60–80 seconds rest, 4 sets.

SESSION 5 HIIT, STAND-ALONE EXERCISES

1 Squat jump »
20 seconds work, 45–60 seconds rest, 8 sets.

2 Burpee/Down and up »
20 seconds work, 45–60 seconds rest, 8 sets.

3 Side-lying open »
20 seconds work, 45–60 seconds rest, 8 sets.

DAY OFF

8-WEEK TRAINING PLAN WEEK 4

SESSION 1 HIIT, STAND-ALONE EXERCISES

1 Running on the spot »
20 seconds work, 45–60 seconds rest, 8 sets.

2 Speed walk-out press-ups »
20 seconds work, 45–60 seconds rest, 8 sets.

3 Rotational chop »
20 seconds work, 45–60 seconds rest, 8 sets.

SESSION 2 RESISTANCE, FULL BODY, STAND-ALONE EXERCISES

1 Incline press-up/Press-up/Kneeling press-up »
10 reps, 60–80 seconds rest, 3 sets.

2 Bodyweight squat »
10 reps, 60–80 seconds rest, 3 sets.

3 Bodyweight bench dip (use a bench, box or chair) »
10 reps, 60–80 seconds rest, 3 sets.

4 Walking lunge/Forward lunge »
10 reps, 60–80 seconds rest, 3 sets.

DAY OFF

SESSION 3 HIIT, STAND-ALONE EXERCISES

1 Side-to-side hops »
20 seconds work, 45–60 seconds rest, 8 sets.

2 Mountain climber/Hop forwards and backwards on the spot »
20 seconds work, 45–60 seconds rest, 8 sets.

3 Skier swing »
20 seconds work, 45–60 seconds rest, 8 sets.

SESSION 4 RESISTANCE, STAND-ALONE EXERCISES, TEMPO 3.1.3

1 Step-up (use a box, chair or bench) »
10 reps (5 each side), 60–80 seconds rest, 3 sets.

2 Narrow hand placement press-up/Kneeling narrow hand placement press-up/Narrow hand placement wall press-up »
10 reps, 60–80 seconds rest, 3 sets.

3 Sumo squat »
10 reps, 60–80 seconds rest, 3 sets.

4 Glute bridge »
10 reps, 60–80 seconds rest, 3 sets.

SESSION 5 HIIT, STAND-ALONE EXERCISES

1 Broad jump to backward hop »
20 seconds work, 45–60 seconds rest, 8 sets.

2 Front plank/Front plank with hand tap »
20 seconds work, 45–60 seconds rest, 8 sets.

3 Star jump »
20 seconds work, 45–60 seconds rest, 8 sets.

DAY OFF

You have now completed the first four weeks of the 8-week training plan. If you feel it would be of benefit, you can repeat this section for another 4–8 weeks before moving on to the second half of the plan. You would do this if you are super-new to training or really out of shape, or to develop better techniques on the suggested exercises.

The next four weeks prepare you in greater depth for the full 12-week programme. They progress slowly, and involve two gym sessions, so you must have access to standard gym equipment.

In addition, there are three HIIT sessions, all of which can be home-based. If you decide to start going to a gym, you can do one of the HIIT exercises on a standard piece of cardio equipment, such as a treadmill, cross-trainer, spin bike or whatever you fancy. You will then just run, cycle or row hard for the amount of time specified in the original exercise.

During this week's work you will notice the move from stand-alone sessions to supersets of exercises. This means that you perform exercise a, then move straight on to exercise b without resting. Once you have completed b, you take your rest, then return to exercise a and go round again for the allotted number of sets.

Note too that the tempo of some resistance exercises has changed.

The next four weeks also see the introduction of HIIT circuits. This means that rather than doing eight sets of one exercise before you move on to the next eight sets, you do one exercise after the other, then take your rest. You then repeat them all again in this way for eight sets.

As in the first four weeks, you are given two days off per week. You can, however, use one of those days off to perform an extra session if you want. Choose one of the HIIT sessions, LISS sessions (see page 74) or resistance sessions from some point in the week and repeat as specified.

PLEASE NOTE
Do not do the same training session twice in a row.
You must take one of your days off to rest and recover.

SESSION 1 HIIT, STAND-ALONE EXERCISES

1 Boxing forwards and upwards while running on spot ››
20 seconds work, 45–60 seconds rest, 8 sets.

2 Carioca ››
20 seconds work, 45–60 seconds rest, 8 sets.

3 Squat jump/Box jump ››
20 seconds work, 45–60 seconds rest, 8 sets.

SESSION 2 RESISTANCE, FULL BODY, SUPERSET, TEMPO 4.1.4

1a Barbell back squat/Dumbbell squat »

6–10 reps, go straight on to exercise 1b.

1b Swiss ball hamstring pull/Machine hamstring curl »

6–10 reps, 60–80 seconds rest, 3 sets, return to exercise 1a after rest.

2a Dumbbell bench press/ Dumbbell fly »

6–10 reps, go straight on to exercise 2b.

2b Barbell bent-over row/Dumbbell bent-over row/Prone row »

6–10 reps, 60–80 seconds rest, 3 sets, return to exercise 2a after rest.

3a Chin-up/Counterweight chin-up/ Lateral pull-down machine »

6–10 reps, go straight on to exercise 3b.

3b Bodyweight dip/Counterweight dip/ Tricep rope push-down »

6–10 reps, 60–80 seconds rest, 3 sets, return to exercise 3a after rest.

SESSION 3 HIIT, CIRCUITS

1 Treadmill run/Other cardio equipment run »

25 seconds work, no rest, go straight to next exercise.

2 Burpee/Down and up »

25 seconds work, no rest, go straight to next exercise.

3 Press-up/Kneeling press-up/ Wall press up »

25 seconds work, no rest, go straight to next exercise.

4 Diagonal rotational chop »

25 seconds work. Rest for 2 minutes post finishing the entire circuit. Perform 4–6 complete circuits.

SESSION 4 RESISTANCE, FULL BODY, SUPERSET, TEMPO 4.1.4

1a Deadlifts/Trap bar deadlift (lifting and lowering phase) »

6–10 reps, go straight on to exercise 1b.

1b Leg extension »

6–10 reps, 60–80 seconds rest, 3 sets, return to exercise 1a after rest.

2a Incline dumbbell press/Incline dumbbell fly »

6–10 reps, go straight on to exercise 2b.

2b Single-arm dumbbell row/Machine row/Cable row »

6–10 reps, 60–80 seconds rest, 3 sets, return to exercise 2a after rest.

3a Barbell upright row/Kettlebell upright row »

6–10 reps, go straight on to exercise 3b.

3b Curl to press/Seated curl to press »

6–10 reps, 60–80 seconds rest, 3 sets, return to exercise 3a after rest.

SESSION 5 HIIT, CIRCUITS

1 Boxing while running on the spot »

25 seconds work, no rest, go straight to next exercise.

2 Spiderman mountain climber »

25 seconds work, no rest, go straight to next exercise.

3 Squat to a box, then jump »

25 seconds work, no rest, go straight to next exercise.

4 Side-lying opens »

25 seconds work, rest for 2 minutes post finishing the entire circuit. Perform 4–6 complete circuits.

DAY OFF

8-WEEK TRAINING PLAN WEEK 6

SESSION 1 HIIT, STAND-ALONE

1 Running on the spot butt kick »

25 seconds work, 45–60 seconds rest, 8 sets.

2 Skater jump »

25 seconds work, 45–60 seconds rest, 8 sets.

3 Mountain climber »

25 seconds work, 45–60 seconds rest, 8 sets.

SESSION 2 RESISTANCE, FULL BODY, SUPERSET, TEMPO 4.1.4

1a Barbell back squat/Dumbbell squat »

6–10 reps, go straight on to exercise 1b.

1b Swiss ball hamstring pull/Machine hamstring curl »

6–10 reps, 60–80 seconds rest, 3 sets, return to exercise 1a after rest.

2a Dumbbell bench press/Dumbbell fly »

6–10 reps, go straight on to exercise 2b.

2b Barbell bent-over row/Dumbbell bent-over row/Prone row »

6–10 reps, 60–80 seconds rest, 3 sets, return to exercise 2a after rest.

3a Chin-up/Counterweight chin-up/Lateral pull-down machine »

6–10 reps, go straight on to exercise 3b.

3b Bodyweight dip/Bodyweight bench dip/Counterweight dip on machine/Tricep rope push-down »

6–10 reps, 60–80 seconds rest, 3 sets, return to exercise 3a after rest.

SESSION 3 HIIT, STAND-ALONE

1 Wattbike/Cross-trainer/VersaClimber/Cardio equipment run »

25 seconds work, 45–60 seconds rest, 8 sets.

2 Dumbbell thruster »

25 seconds work, 45–60 seconds rest, 8 sets.

3 Lunge change-up/Walking lunge »

25 seconds work, 45–60 seconds rest, 8 sets.

SESSION 4 RESISTANCE, FULL BODY, SUPERSET

1a Deadlift/Trap bar deadlift (lifting and lowering phase) »

6–10 reps, go straight on to exercise 1b.

1b Leg extension »

6–10 reps, 60–80 seconds rest, 3 sets, return to exercise 1a after rest.

2a Incline dumbbell press »

6–10 reps, go straight on to exercise 2b.

2b Single-arm dumbbell row/Machine row/Cable row »

6–10 reps, 60–80 seconds rest, 3 sets, return to exercise 1a after rest.

3a Barbell upright row/Kettlebell upright row »

6–10 reps, go straight on to exercise 3b.

3b Curl to press »

6–10 reps, 60–80 seconds rest, 3 sets, return to exercise 3a after rest.

SESSION 5 HIIT, CIRCUITS

1 Burpee/Down and up »

25 seconds work, no rest, go straight to next exercise.

2 Backwards and forward shuttle »

25 seconds work, no rest, go straight to next exercise.

3 Diagonal rotational chop »

25 seconds work, no rest, go straight to next exercise.

4 Decline press-up/Normal press-up/Kneeling press-up »

25 seconds work, rest for 2 minutes post finishing the entire circuit. Perform 4–6 complete circuits.

DAY OFF

8-WEEK TRAINING PLAN WEEK 7

SESSION 1 HIIT, STAND-ALONE EXERCISES

1 Boxing forwards and upwards while running on the spot »

20 seconds work, 45–60 seconds rest, 8 sets.

2 Side-to-side shuffle »

20 seconds work, 45–60 seconds rest, 8 sets.

3 Squat jump/Box jump »

20 seconds work, 45–60 seconds rest, 8 sets.

SESSION 2 RESISTANCE FULL BODY, SUPERSET, TEMPO 4.1.4

1a Barbell back squat/Dumbbell squat »

6–10 reps, go straight to exercise 1b.

1b Swiss ball hamstring pulls/Machine hamstring curl »

6–10 reps, 60–80 seconds rest, 3 sets, return to exercise 1a after rest.

2a Dumbbell bench press/Dumbbell fly »

6–10 reps, go straight to exercise 2b.

2b Barbell bent-over row/Dumbbell bent-over row/Prone row »

6–10 reps, 60–80 seconds rest, 3 sets, return to exercise 2a after rest.

3a Chin-up/Counterweight chin-up/Lateral pull-down »

6–10 reps, go straight on to exercise 3b.

3b Bodyweight dip/Tricep rope push-down/Counterweight dip »

6–10 reps, 60–80 seconds rest, 3 sets, return to exercise 3a after rest.

SESSION 3 HIIT, CIRCUITS

1 Treadmill run/Other cardio equipment run »

25 seconds work, no rest, go straight to next exercise.

2 Burpee/Down and up »

25 seconds work, no rest, go straight to next exercise.

3 Press-up/Kneeling press-up/Wall press-up »

25 seconds work, no rest, go straight to next exercise.

4 Diagonal rotational chop »

25 seconds work, rest for 2 minutes post finishing the entire circuit. Perform 4–6 complete circuits.

SESSION 4 RESISTANCE, FULL BODY, SUPERSET, TEMPO 4.1.4

1a Deadlift/Trap bar deadlift (lifting and lowering phase) »

6–10 reps, go straight on to exercise 1b.

1b Leg extension »

6–10 reps, 60–80 seconds rest, 3 sets, return to exercise 1a after rest.

2a Incline dumbbell press/Incline dumbbell fly »

6–10 reps, go straight on to exercise 2b.

2b Single-arm dumbbell row/Machine row/Cable row »

6–10 reps, 60–80 seconds rest, 3 sets, return to exercise 2a after rest.

3a Barbell upright row/ Kettle bell upright row »

6–10 reps, go straight on to exercise 3b.

3b Curl to press »

6–10 reps, 60–80 seconds rest, 3 sets, return to exercise 3a after rest.

SESSION 5 HIIT, CIRCUITS

1 Skipping with a rope on the spot/Skipping without a rope on the spot »

25 seconds work, no rest, go straight on to next exercise.

2 Spiderman mountain climber »

25 seconds work, no rest, go straight on to next exercise.

3 Squat to box jump/Squat jump »

25 seconds work, no rest, go straight on to next exercise.

4 Side-lying opens »

25 seconds work, rest for 2 minutes post finishing the entire circuit. Perform 4–6 complete circuits.

DAY OFF

8-WEEK TRAINING PLAN WEEK 8

SESSION 1 HIIT, STAND-ALONE

1 Running on the spot butt kick »
25 seconds work, 45–60 seconds rest, 8 sets.

2 Skater jump »
25 seconds work, 45–60 seconds rest, 8 sets.

3 Mountain climber »
25 seconds work, 45–60 seconds rest, 8 sets.

SESSION 2 RESISTANCE, FULL BODY, SUPERSET, TEMPO 4.1.4

1a Barbell back squat/Dumbbell squat »
6–10 reps, go straight on to exercise 1b.

1b Swiss ball hamstring pull/Machine hamstring curl »
6–10 reps, 60–80 seconds rest, 3 sets, return to exercise 1a after rest.

2a Dumbbell bench press/Dumbbell fly »
6–10 reps, go straight on to exercise 2b.

2b Barbell bent-over row/Dumbbell bent-over row/Prone row »
6–10 reps, 60–80 seconds rest, 3 sets, return to exercise 2a after rest.

3a Chin-up/Counterweight chin-up/Lateral pull-down »
10 reps, go straight on to exercise 3b.

3b Bodyweight dip/Tricep rope push-down/Counterweight dip »
6–10 reps, 60–80 seconds rest, 3 sets, return to exercise 3a after rest.

SESSION 3 HIIT, STAND-ALONE EXERCISES

1 Wattbike/Cross-trainer/VersaClimber/Cardio equipment run »
25 seconds work, 45–60 seconds rest, 8 sets.

2 Dumbbell thruster »
25 seconds work, 45–60 seconds rest, 8 sets.

3 Lunge change-up/Walking lunge »
25 seconds work, 45–60 seconds rest, 8 sets.

SESSION 4 RESISTANCE, FULL BODY, SUPERSET

1a Deadlift/Trap bar deadlift (lifting and lowering phase) »
6–10 reps, go straight on to exercise 1b.

1b Leg extension »
6–10 reps, 60–80 seconds rest, 3 sets, return to exercise 1a after rest.

2a Incline dumbbell press/Incline dumbbell fly »
6–10 reps, go straight on to exercise 2b.

2b Machine row/Cable row/Prone row »
6–10 reps, 60–80 seconds rest, 3 sets, return to exercise 2a after rest.

3a Barbell upright row/Kettlebell row »
6–10 reps, go straight on to exercise 3b.

3b Curl to press »
6–10 reps, 60–80 seconds rest, 3 sets, return to exercise 3a after rest.

SESSION 5 HIIT, CIRCUITS

1 Burpee/Down and up »
25 seconds work, no rest, go straight on to next exercise.

2 Backwards and forwards shuttle »
25 seconds work, no rest, go straight on to next exercise.

3 Diagonal rotational chop »
25 seconds work, no rest, go straight on to next exercise.

4 Decline press-up/Normal press-up/Kneeling press-up »
25 seconds work, rest for 2 minutes post finishing the entire circuit. Perform 4–6 complete circuits.

DAY OFF

Congratulations! You have finished the 8-week beginner's training programme. This will have set you up nicely for the full 12-week programme that follows, so when you are ready, you can get cracking on changing your body forever.

If you have found benefit in doing the 8-week programme, or feel you need more time to get used to the exercises, that's no problem – you can repeat it as many times as you like until you are ready to move on. Those who have never really trained before, or those who need to lose a lot of weight, could find it especially beneficial to retrace their steps.

12-WEEK TRAINING PLAN

For this plan you need access to a gym in order to do the exercises properly and get the best results.

HOW TO USE THE PLAN

As we are all different, I believe that training should be individualised – one shoe does not fit all. I have therefore structured this programme with that in mind, but there are three ways in which it can be approached.

>> **If your goal is simply to build muscle,** you need to be doing 4–5 resistance sessions per week and one HIIT session per week. Depending on how you feel, you can use your days off to perform HIIT or LISS top-ups. However, if you are doing the resistance sessions properly, you will be pretty sore, so will need to take a rest.

>> **If you want to lose fat and build muscle,** you need to perform two HITT sessions and three resistance sessions per week. Then, if you feel the need to do more work, you can use your day off to perform an extra HIIT, LISS or resistance session.

>> **If you simply want to lose weight,** perform three HIIT sessions, one LISS session and one resistance session per week. If you feel the need to do more work, you can perform more cardio, either HIIT or LISS, on one of your days off. Remember, though, that it's important to take at least one day off.

Opposite is a weekly timetable that shows how your training week might look. The sessions can be done morning, afternoon or evening – whatever time of day suits you.

SUMMARY OF THE 12-WEEK PLAN

Here is an overview of how the 12 weeks look in term of intensity:

Week 1	>>	Build-up
Week 2	>>	Medium intensity
Weeks 3–6	>>	High intensity
Week 7	>>	Medium intensity
Weeks 8–12	>>	High intensity

It is important to note that training does not have to finish after week 12. I recommend that you rest for a week, then start the process again, making the programme 24 weeks long. Or if you want a new challenge you can try something different. Remember, it's not possible to try and achieve the goals of being big, fit, strong and powerful all in one go, you need to choose another goal and stick with it for a period of time. I suggest you take a week off and think about what you want to achieve next. Maybe you'd like to get slightly leaner, in which case you can repeat the 8-week plan. Or perhaps you want to build more muscle, in which case you can try my *Lean Gains*

WEEKLY PLAN FOR **WEIGHT LOSS**

	MON	TUES	WEDS	THURS	FRI	SAT	SUN
am or pm	HIIT	Resistance	Day off or optional training	HIIT	LISS	HIIT	Day off or optional training

WEEKLY PLAN FOR **WEIGHT LOSS AND MUSCLE BUILDING**

	MON	TUES	WEDS	THURS	FRI	SAT	SUN
am or pm	HIIT	Resistance	Day off or optional training	HIIT	Resistance or optional training	Day off	Resistance

WEEKLY PLAN FOR **MUSCLE BUILDING**

	MON	TUES	WEDS	THURS	FRI	SAT	SUN
am or pm	HIIT	Resistance	Day off or optional training	HIIT	LISS	HITT	Resistance or optional training

ebook (www.jameshaskell.com/learn-more-lean-gains) or repeat the 12-week section of this plan, as you will get different results if you follow it in different ways. Alternatively, you can find a completely different plan to follow. Remember you are training for life, not just for 12 weeks.

CHOOSE A WEIGHT TO START LIFTING

Everyone following this 12-week plan will be at a different level of fitness, ability and strength, so it would not be sensible for me to suggest a weight that you can start lifting. Here are some tips on the best way to choose your weight.

>> **Select a weight that you find manageable** simply by picking it up and trying it. Your warm-up is a good time for this. If you then do a lifting set and find it doesn't stress you at all, mark it down as a warm-up and choose a heavier weight. The point is to work hard, not just tick boxes and go through the motions.

>> **If you are aiming to do 10 reps** and you find the last two fairly hard, the weight you have chosen is a good place to start. Ideally, you should find it hard to do the last 2–3 reps of any working set. Use your chosen weight for the next set, but when you come to do the workout again, increase the weight by a margin of 3–5 per cent.

>> **If you get to six reps in a session** and you can't lift again, or you aren't able to finish the remaining sets, you have gone too heavy too soon. You need to drop the weight and make that your starting point for the next session.

>> **German volume training is a bit different.** As this form of training requires 10 sets of 10 reps, or 10 sets of 6–8 reps, you want to begin with a weight you could lift for 20 reps, possibly to failure (by which I mean you couldn't lift it at all for another rep). For most people on most exercises, that weight would represent 65 per cent of their one rep maximum load. This might seem a bit complicated, but through trial and error you will get it right. For example, if my one rep max on bench press is 100kg, I would start my first set of 10 reps on 65kg. It's important that you get through the full number of sets, so you can't afford to go too heavy too early or you will fall short.

It's now time to start training. The tables above tells you the number and type of sessions you should be doing. As you work through the 12-week plan, any key changes are noted at the beginning of each week. These include rest times, tempo, number of sets and weights.

>> **Remember to do a warm-up routine** before every workout session (see page 45).

>> **Days off** – you have the option to fully rest, but if you prefer, you can do a LISS session (see page 174), or perform another HIIT or resistance session, depending on what your goal is, how you feel and the results you want to get. Do remember, though, that recovery is very important. Please refer to the recovery and mobility advice in Chapter 5 (see page 149), where various options – ice baths, foam rolling, compression garments and so forth – are discussed.

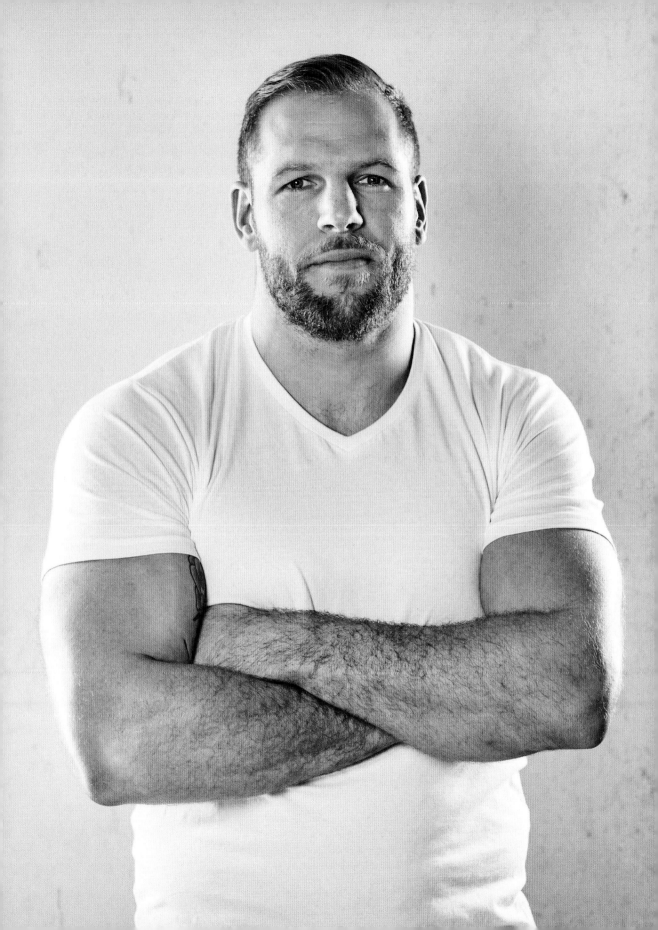

Once you have chosen your goal, you will understand what sessions you need to be doing. Each day will include either a resistance session or a HIIT session. If you want to add a LISS workout, see page 174.

SESSION 1 RESISTANCE LOWER BODY, STAND-ALONE EXERCISES, TEMPO 4.1.4

1 Barbell back squat/Dumbbell squat »

10 reps, 60–80 seconds rest, 5 sets.

2 Swiss ball hamstring pull/Machine hamstring curl »

10 reps, 60–80 seconds rest, 5 sets.

3 Deadlift/Trap bar deadlift (raising and lowering phase) »

10 reps, 60–80 seconds rest, 3 sets.

4 Calf-raise/Machine-assisted calf-raise »

10 reps, 60–80 seconds rest, 3 sets.

SESSION 1 HIIT, CIRCUITS

1 Boxing while running on the spot »

25 seconds work, no rest, go straight on to next exercise.

2 Mountain climber »

25 seconds work, no rest, go straight on to next exercise.

3 Running on and off a low box »

25 seconds work, no rest, go straight on to next exercise.

4 Side-lying open »

25 seconds work, rest for 2 minutes post finishing the entire circuit. Perform 5–8 complete circuits.

SESSION 2 RESISTANCE UPPER BODY, STAND-ALONE EXERCISES, TEMPO 4.1.4

1 Dumbbell bench press/Dumbbell fly/Machine press »

10 reps, 60–80 seconds rest, 5 sets.

2 Barbell bent-over row/Dumbbell bent-over row/Prone row »

10 reps, 60–80 seconds rest, 5 sets.

3 Military press/Seated shoulder press »

10 reps, 60–80 seconds rest, 3 sets.

4 Chin-up/Counterweight chin-up/Lateral pull-down »

10 reps, 60–80 seconds rest, 3 sets.

5 Bodyweight dip/Weighted dip/Counterweight dip/Tricep rope pull-down »

10 reps, 60–80 seconds rest, 3 sets.

SESSION 2 HIIT, STAND-ALONE EXERCISES

1 Spin bike/Wattbike/Cross-trainer/VersaClimber (or any piece of cardio equipment) »

25 seconds work, 45–60 seconds rest, 8 sets.

2 Dumbbell thruster »

25 seconds work, 45–60 seconds rest, 8 sets.

3 Lunge change-up/Walking lunge »

25 seconds work, 45–60 seconds rest, 8 sets.

DAY OFF

SESSION 3 RESISTANCE LOWER BODY, STAND-ALONE EXERCISES, TEMPO 4.1.4

1 Barbell front squat/Goblet squat »

10 reps, 60–80 seconds rest, 5 sets.

2 Glute bridge »

10 reps, 60–80 seconds rest, 5 sets.

3 Walking lunge/Forward lunge »

10 reps each side, 60–80 seconds rest, 2 sets.

4 Calf-raise/Machine-assisted calf-raise »

20 reps, 60–80 seconds rest, 2 sets.

SESSION 3 HIIT, STAND-ALONE EXERCISES

1 Squat jump »

20 seconds work, 45–60 seconds rest, 8 sets.

2 Burpee/Down and up »

20 seconds work, 45–60 seconds rest, 8 sets.

3 Front plank »

20 seconds work, 45–60 seconds rest, 8 sets.

SESSION 4 RESISTANCE UPPER BODY, STAND-ALONE EXERCISES, TEMPO 4.1.4

1 Incline dumbbell press/Incline dumbbell fly/Machine press »

10 reps, 60–80 seconds rest, 5 sets.

2 Single-arm dumbbell row/Machine row/Cable row »

10 reps, 60–80 seconds rest, 5 sets.

3 Barbell upright row/Dumbbell upright row/Kettlebell row »

10 reps, 60–80 seconds rest, 5 sets.

4 EZ bar curl/Barbell curl/Dumbbell curl »

12–15 reps, 60–80 seconds rest, 2 sets.

5 Tricep rope push-down »

12–15 reps, 60–80 seconds rest, 2 sets.

SESSION 4 HIIT, STAND-ALONE EXERCISES

1 Side-to-side hop »

20 seconds work, 45–60 seconds rest, 8 sets.

2 Mountain climber »

20 seconds work, 45–60 seconds rest, 8 sets.

3 Skier swing »

20 seconds work, 45–60 seconds rest, 8 sets.

SESSION 5 RESISTANCE FULL BODY, SUPERSET, TEMPO 4.1.4

1a Bulgarian split squat »

10 reps each side, go straight on to exercise 1b.

1b Hamstring extension/Romanian deadlift »

10 reps, 60–80 seconds rest, return to exercise 1a. Perform 3 complete sets.

2a Cable face-pull »

10 reps, move straight on to exercise 2b.

2b Single-arm dumbbell row/Machine row/Cable row »

10 reps, 60–80 seconds rest, return to exercise 2a. Perform 3 complete sets.

3a Seated hammer curl »

10 reps, move straight on to exercise 3b.

3b Close-grip bench press/Narrow hand placement tricep press ups »

10 reps, 60–80 seconds rest, return to exercise 3a. Perform 3 complete sets.

SESSION 5 HIIT, STAND-ALONE EXERCISES

1 Broad jump to backward hop »

20 seconds work, 45–60 seconds, 8 sets.

2 Front plank with hand tap/Front plank »

20 seconds work, 45–60 seconds, 8 sets.

3 Star jump »

20 seconds work, 45–60 seconds, 8 sets.

DAY OFF

Please note the following changes during this week:
>> The rest period changes slightly for exercises with 8 sets. You will be resting for 90 seconds.
>> With supersets, you normally perform exercises a and b before taking a rest. In this section, some supersets require you to rest after performing each exercise, and to perform the allotted number of sets in the same way. Make sure you read the instructions accurately.
>> The tempo for a number of exercises changes to 4.1.2, so please look out for these.

SESSION 1 RESISTANCE LOWER BODY, SUPERSET, TEMPO 4.1.2

1a Barbell back squat/Dumbbell squat >>

10 reps, 90 seconds rest, go straight on to exercise 1b.

1b Swiss ball hamstring pull/Machine hamstring curl >>

10 reps, rest 90 seconds, return to exercise 1a. Perform 8 complete sets.

2a Deadlift/Trap bar deadlift >>

10 reps, rest 90 seconds, go straight on to exercise b

2b Calf-raise/Machine-assisted calf-raise >>

10 reps, 90 seconds rest, return to exercise 2a. Perform 4 complete sets.

SESSION 1 HIIT, CIRCUITS

1 Running on the spot with high knees >>

20 seconds work, no rest, go straight on to next exercise.

2 Bodyweight squat >>

20 seconds work, no rest, go straight on to next exercise.

3 Burpee/Down and up >>

20 seconds work, no rest, go straight on to next exercise.

4 Mountain climber/Hop forwards and backwards on the spot >>

20 seconds work, 2 minutes rest post finishing the entire circuit. Perform 4–6 complete circuits.

SESSION 2 RESISTANCE UPPER BODY, SUPERSET/STAND-ALONE EXERCISES, TEMPO 4.1.2

1a Dumbbell bench press/Dumbbell fly >>

10 reps, 90 seconds rest, go straight on to exercise 1b.

1b Barbell bent-over row/Dumbbell bent-over row/Prone row >>

10 reps, 90 seconds rest, return to exercise 1a. Perform 8 complete sets.

2 Military press/Shoulder press >>

10 reps, 60–80 seconds rest, 4 sets.

3a Chin-up/Counterweight chin-up/Lateral pull-down >>

10 reps, go straight on to exercise 3b.

3b Bodyweight dip/Weighted dip/Tricep rope push-down >>

10 reps, 60–80 seconds rest, return to exercise 3a. Perform 4 complete sets.

SESSION 2 HIIT, STAND-ALONE EXERCISES

1 Running on the spot »
20 seconds work, 45–60 seconds rest, 8 sets.

2 Star jump »
20 seconds work, 45–60 seconds rest, 8 sets.

3 Jumping mountain climber »
20 seconds work, 45–60 seconds rest, 8 sets.

DAY OFF

SESSION 3 RESISTANCE LOWER BODY, SUPERSET, TEMPO 4.1.2

1a Barbell front squat/Goblet squat »
10 reps, 90 seconds rest, go straight on to exercise 1b.

1b Forward lunge »
10 reps, 90 seconds rest, return to exercise 1a. Perform 8 complete sets.

2a Glute bridge »
10 reps, 60–80 seconds rest, go straight on to exercise 2b.

2b Calf-raise/Machine-assisted calf-raise »
10 reps, 60–80 seconds rest, return to exercise 2a. Perform 4 complete sets.

SESSION 3 HIIT, STAND-ALONE EXERCISES

1 Running on the spot with tuck jumps »
20 seconds work, 45–60 seconds rest, 8 sets.

2 Side-to-side hop »
20 seconds work, 45–60 seconds rest, 8 sets.

3 Speed walkouts to press-up »
20 seconds work, 45–60 seconds rest, 8 sets.

SESSION 4 RESISTANCE UPPER BODY, SUPERSET/STAND-ALONE EXERCISES, TEMPO 4.1.2

1a Incline dumbbell press/Dumbbell fly/Machine press »
10 reps, 90 seconds rest, go straight on to exercise 1b.

1b Seated cable row/Machine row/Prone row »
10 reps, 90 seconds rest, return to exercise 1a. Perform 8 complete sets.

2 Barbell upright row/Kettlebell upright row »
10 reps, 60–80 seconds rest, 4 sets.

3a EZ bar curl/Barbell curl »
10 reps, 60–80 seconds rest, go straight on to exercise 3b.

3b Tricep rope push-down »
10 reps, 60–80 seconds rest, return to exercise 3a. Perform 4 complete sets.

SESSION 4 HIIT, CIRCUITS

1 Treadmill run/Other cardio equipment run »
25 seconds work, no rest, go straight on to next exercise.

2 Burpee/Down and up »
25 seconds work, no rest, go straight on to next exercise.

3 Dive-bomber press-up/Normal press-up »
25 seconds work, rest for 2 minutes post finishing the entire circuit. Perform 4–6 complete circuits.

12-WEEK TRAINING PLAN WEEK 2

SESSION 5 RESISTANCE FULL BODY, SUPERSET, TEMPO 4.1.2

1a Bulgarian split squat »

10 reps each side, 60–80 seconds rest, go straight on to exercise 1b.

1b Hamstring extension/Romanian deadlift »

10 reps, 60–80 seconds rest, return to exercise 1a. Perform 4 complete sets.

2a Cable face-pull »

10 reps each side, 60–80 seconds rest, go straight on to exercise 2b.

2b Single-arm dumbbell row/ Cable row/Machine row »

10 reps, 60–80 seconds rest, return to exercise 2a, perform 4 complete sets.

3a Seated hammer curl »

10 reps each side, 60–80 seconds rest, go straight on to exercise 3b.

3b Close-grip bench press/Narrow hand placement press-up »

10 reps, 60–80 seconds rest, return to exercise 3a. Perform 4 complete sets.

SESSION 5 HIIT, CIRCUITS

1 Boxing while running on the spot »

25 seconds work, no rest, go straight on to next exercise.

2 Mountain climber »

25 seconds work, no rest, go straight on to next exercise.

3 Seal jack »

25 seconds work, no rest, go straight on to next exercise.

4 Side-lying opens »

25 seconds work, rest for 2 minutes post finishing the entire circuit. Perform 4–6 complete circuits.

DAY OFF

This is our first week of super-high-intensity training within the 12-week programme. Please note the following changes:

>> Here we introduce German volume work, which consists of 10 sets of 10 reps.

>> The tempo changes for some exercises, as follows: 4 seconds lowering, 1 second pause, 1 second raise. It is written 4.1.1.

>> Rest for certain sections and exercises is set at 90 seconds.

This part of the training programme will really push you to your limits. As mentioned on page 31, you must avoid over-training, and it's important to listen to your body. Do remember, though, that sore muscles are to be expected. Make sure you take the time to recover as best you can.

Whatever goal you have chosen – weight loss, body fat reduction and muscle building, or just muscle building – the training programme can be approached in three different ways:

1 Do all the sessions as prescribed, which means performing five sessions a week and using the days off for rest and recovery.

2 Choose the three main sessions of the week – lower body, upper body or full body – then perform two HIIT or LISS sessions on your days off, or extra resistance sessions.

3 Perform three HIIT sessions and two resistance sessions for lower body and upper body. Then, on your days off, you can decide to perform more resistance training, a LISS session or another HIIT circuit.

SESSION 1 RESISTANCE LOWER BODY, SUPERSET, TEMPO 4.1.1

1a Barbell back squat/Dumbbell squat »

10 reps, 90 seconds rest, go straight on to exercise 1b.

1b Swiss ball hamstring pulls/ Machine hamstring curl »

10 reps, 90 seconds rest, return to exercise 1a. Perform 10 complete sets.

2a Deadlift/Trap bar deadlift »

10 reps, 60–80 seconds rest, go straight on to exercise 2b.

2b Calf-raise/Machine-assisted calf-raise »

10 reps, 90 seconds rest, return to exercise 2a. Perform 6 complete sets.

SESSION 1 HIIT, STAND-ALONE EXERCISES

1 Running on the spot butt kick »

25 seconds work, 45–60 seconds rest, 8 sets.

2 Skater jump »

25 seconds work, 45–60 seconds rest, 8 sets.

3 Jumping mountain climber »

25 seconds work, 45–60 seconds rest, 8 sets.

12-WEEK TRAINING PLAN WEEK 3

SESSION 2 RESISTANCE UPPER BODY, SUPERSET, TEMPO 4.1.1

1a Dumbbell bench press/ Dumbbell fly/Machine press »

10 reps, 90 seconds rest, go straight on to exercise 1b.

1b Barbell bent-over row/Dumbbell bent-over row/Prone row »

10 reps, 90 seconds rest, return to exercise 1a. Perform 10 complete sets of this.

2 Military press/Shoulder press/ Seated shoulder press »

10 reps, 60–80 seconds rest, 6 sets.

3a Chin-up/Counterweight chin-up/ Lateral pull-down »

10 reps, go straight on to exercise 3b.

3b Bodyweight dip/Counterweight dip/Bench dip/Tricep rope push-down »

10 reps, 60–80 seconds rest, return to exercise 3a. Perform 6 complete sets.

SESSION 2 HIIT, STAND-ALONE EXERCISES

1 Boxing forwards and upwards while running on the spot »

25 seconds work, 45–60 seconds rest, 8 sets.

2 Carioca »

25 seconds work, 45–60 seconds rest, 8 sets.

3 Squat jump »

20 seconds work, 45–60 seconds rest, 8 sets.

DAY OFF

SESSION 3 RESISTANCE LOWER BODY, SUPERSET, TEMPO 4.1.1

1a Barbell front squat/Goblet squat »

10 reps, 90 seconds rest, go straight on to exercise 1b.

1b Walking lunge/Forward lunge »

10 reps, rest 90 seconds, return to exercise 1a. Perform 10 complete sets.

2a Glute bridge »

10 reps, 60–80 seconds rest, go straight on to exercise 2b.

2b Calf-raise/Machine-assisted calf-raise »

10 reps, 60–80 seconds rest, return to exercise 2a. Perform 6 complete sets.

SESSION 3 HIIT, CIRCUITS

1 Burpee/Down and up »

25 seconds work, no rest, go straight on to next exercise.

2 Forwards and backwards shuttle »

25 seconds work, no rest, go straight on to next exercise.

3 Diagonal rotational chop »

25 seconds work, no rest, go straight on to next exercise.

4 Decline press-up/Normal press-up/ Kneeling press-up »

25 seconds work. Rest for 2 minutes post finishing the entire circuit. Perform 4–6 complete circuits.

SESSION 4 RESISTANCE UPPER BODY, SUPERSET, TEMPO 4.1.4

1a Incline dumbbell press/Incline dumbbell fly/Machine press »

10 reps, 90 seconds rest, go straight on to exercise 1b.

1b Single-arm dumbbell row/Seated cable row/Machine row »

10 reps, 90 seconds rest, return to exercise 1a. Perform 10 complete sets.

2 Barbell upright row/Kettlebell upright row »

10 reps, 60–80 seconds rest, 6 sets.

3a EZ bar curl/Barbell curl/ Dumbbell curl »

10 reps, 60–80 seconds rest, go straight on to exercise 3b.

3b Tricep rope push-down »

10 reps, 60–80 seconds rest, return to exercise 3a. Perform 6 complete sets.

SESSION 4 HIIT, STAND-ALONE EXERCISES

1 Treadmill run/Other cardio equipment sprint »

25 seconds work, 45–60 seconds rest, 8 sets.

2 Drop squat »

25 seconds work, 45–60 seconds rest, 8 sets.

3 Side-to-side hop »

25 seconds work, 45–60 seconds rest, 8 sets.

SESSION 5 RESISTANCE FULL BODY, SUPERSET, TEMPO 4.1.1

1a Bulgarian split squat »

10 reps each side, 60–80 seconds rest, go straight on to exercise 1b.

1b Hamstring extension/Romanian deadlift »

10 reps, 60–80 seconds rest, return to exercise 1a. Perform 5 complete sets.

2a Cable face-pulls »

10 reps each side, 60–80 seconds rest, go straight on to exercise 2b.

2b Single-arm dumbbell row/ Cable row/Machine row »

10 reps, 60–80 seconds rest, return to exercise 2a. Perform 4 complete sets.

3a Seated hammer curl »

10 reps each side, 60–80 seconds rest, go straight on to exercise 3b.

3b Close-grip bench press/Narrow hand placement press-up »

10 reps, 60–80 seconds rest, return to exercise 3a. Perform 4 complete sets.

SESSION 5 HIIT, STAND-ALONE EXERCISES

1 Boxing forwards and upwards while running on the spot »

25 seconds work, 45–60 seconds rest, 8 sets.

2 Carioca »

25 seconds work, 45–60 seconds rest, 8 sets.

3 Squat jump »

25 seconds work, 45–60 seconds rest, 8 sets.

DAY OFF

12-WEEK TRAINING PLAN WEEK 4

Everything is the same as Week 3 in terms of resistance, rest and tempo, but the HIIT sessions have changed.

SESSION 1
RESISTANCE LOWER BODY, SUPERSET, TEMPO 4.1.1

1a Barbell back squat/Dumbbell squat »

10 reps, 90 seconds rest, go straight on to exercise 1b.

1b Swiss ball hamstring pulls/ Machine hamstring curl »

10 reps, 90 seconds rest, return to exercise 1a. Perform 10 complete sets.

2a Deadlift/Trap bar deadlift »

10 reps, 60–80 seconds rest, go straight on to exercise 2b.

2b Calf-raise/Machine-assisted calf-raise »

10 reps, 90 seconds rest, return to exercise 2a. Perform 6 complete sets.

SESSION 1 HIIT, STAND-ALONE EXERCISES

1 Skipping with rope/Skipping on the spot »

25 seconds work, 45–60 seconds rest, 8 sets.

2 In-and-out squat »

25 seconds work, 45–60 seconds rest, 8 sets.

3 Jumping mountain climber »

25 seconds work, 45–60 seconds rest, 8 sets.

SESSION 2 RESISTANCE UPPER BODY, SUPERSET, TEMPO 4.1.1

1a Dumbbell bench press/ Dumbbell fly/Machine press »

10 reps, 90 seconds rest, go straight on to exercise 1b.

1b Barbell bent-over row/Dumbbell bent-over row/Prone row »

10 reps, 90 seconds rest, return to exercise 1a. Perform 10 complete sets.

2 Military press/Shoulder press/ Seated shoulder press »

10 reps, 60–80 seconds rest, 6 complete sets.

3a Chin-up/Counterweight chin-up/ Lateral pull-down »

10 reps, go straight on to exercise 3b.

3b Bodyweight dip/Counterweight dip/Tricep push-down »

10 reps, 60–80 seconds rest, return to exercise 3a. Perform 6 complete sets.

SESSION 2 HIIT, STAND-ALONE EXERCISES

1 Running on the spot with burpees »

20 seconds work, 45–60 seconds rest, 8 sets.

2 Carioca »

20 seconds work, 45–60 seconds rest, 8 sets.

3 Medicine ball slam/Bodyweight slam »

20 seconds work, 45–60 seconds rest, 8 sets.

DAY OFF

SESSION 3 RESISTANCE LOWER BODY, SUPERSET, TEMPO 4.1.1

1a Barbell front squat/Goblet squat »

10 reps, 90 seconds rest, go straight on to exercise 1b.

1b Walking lunge/Forward lunge »

10 reps, 90 seconds rest, return to exercise 1a. Perform 10 complete sets.

2a Glute bridge »

10 reps, 60–80 seconds rest, go straight on to exercise 2b.

2b Calf-raise/Machine-assisted calf-raise »

10 reps, 60–80 seconds rest, return to exercise 2a. Perform 6 complete sets.

SESSION 3 HIIT, CIRCUITS

1 Burpee/Down and up »

25 seconds work, no rest, go straight on to next exercise.

2 Low rotational chop »

25 seconds work, no rest, go straight on to next exercise.

3 Full body crunch »

25 seconds work, no rest, go straight on to next exercise.

4 Decline press-up/Normal press-up »

25 seconds work. Rest for 2 minutes post finishing the entire circuit. Perform 4–6 complete circuits.

SESSION 4 RESISTANCE UPPER BODY, SUPERSET, TEMPO 4.1.4

1a Incline dumbbell press/Incline dumbbell fly/Machine press »

10 reps, 90 seconds rest, go straight on to exercise 1b.

1b Single-arm dumbbell row/Cable row/Machine row »

10 reps, 90 seconds rest, return to exercise 1a. Perform 10 complete sets.

2 Barbell upright row/Kettlebell row

– 10 reps, 60–80 seconds rest, 6 sets.

3a EZ bar curl/Barbell curl »

10 reps, 60–80 seconds rest, go straight on to exercise 3b.

3b Tricep rope push-down »

10 reps, 60–80 seconds rest, return to exercise 3a. Perform 6 complete sets.

SESSION 4 HIIT, STAND-ALONE EXERCISES

1 Treadmill run/Other cardio equipment run »

25 seconds work, 45–60 seconds rest, 8 sets.

2 Halo slam »

25 seconds work, 45–60 seconds rest, 8 sets.

3 Side-to-side shuffle »

25 seconds work, 45–60 seconds rest, 8 sets.

SESSION 5 RESISTANCE FULL BODY, SUPERSET, TEMPO 4.1.1

1a Bulgarian split squat »

10 reps each side, 60–80 seconds rest, go straight on to exercise 1b.

1b Hamstring extension/Romanian deadlift »

10 reps, 60–80 seconds rest, return to exercise 1a. Perform 5 complete sets.

2a Cable face-pull »

10 reps each side, 60–80 seconds rest, go straight on to exercise 2b.

2b Single-arm dumbbell row/Cable row/Machine row »

10 reps, 60–80 seconds rest, return to exercise 2a. Perform 4 complete sets.

3a Seated hammer curl »

10 reps each side, 60–80 seconds rest, go straight on to exercise 3b.

3b Close-grip bench press/Narrow hand placement press-up »

10 reps, 60–80 seconds rest, return to exercise 3a. Perform 4 complete sets.

SESSION 5 HIIT, STAND-ALONE EXERCISES

1 Star jump »

20 seconds work, 45–60 seconds rest, 8 sets.

2 Carioca side-to-side »

20 seconds work, 45–60 seconds rest, 8 sets.

3 Squat jump »

20 seconds work, 45–60 seconds rest, 8 sets.

DAY OFF

SESSION 1 RESISTANCE LOWER BODY, SUPERSET, TEMPO 4.1.1

1a Barbell back squat/Dumbbell squat »

10 reps, 90 seconds rest, go straight on to exercise 1b.

1b Swiss ball hamstring pull/ Machine hamstring curl »

10 reps, 90 seconds rest, return to exercise 1a. Perform 10 complete sets.

2a Deadlift/Trap bar deadlift »

10 reps, 60–80 seconds rest, go straight on to exercise 2b.

2b Calf-raise/Machine-assisted calf-raise »

10 reps, 90 seconds rest, return to exercise 2a. Perform 6 complete sets.

SESSION 1 HIIT, STAND-ALONE EXERCISES

1 High knees on the spot »

25 seconds work, 45–60 seconds rest, 8 sets.

2 In-and-out squat »

25 seconds work, 45–60 seconds rest, 8 sets.

3 Spiderman mountain climber »

25 seconds work, 45–60 seconds rest, 8 sets.

SESSION 2 RESISTANCE UPPER BODY, SUPERSET, TEMPO 4.1.1

1a Dumbbell bench press/ Dumbbell fly/Machine press »

10 reps, 90 seconds rest, go straight on to exercise 1b.

1b Bent-over row/Dumbbell row/ Prone row »

10 reps, 90 seconds rest, return to exercise 1a. Perform 10 complete sets.

2 Military press/Shoulder press/ Seated shoulder press »

10 reps, 60–80 seconds rest, 6 sets.

3a Chin-up/Counterweight chin-up/ Lateral pull-down »

10 reps, go straight on to exercise 3b.

3b Bodyweight dip/Counterweight dip/Tricep rope push-down »

10 reps, 60–80 seconds rest, return to exercise 3a. Perform 6 complete sets.

SESSION 2 HIIT, STAND-ALONE EXERCISES

1 Boxing forwards and upwards while running on the spot »

25 seconds work, 45–60 seconds rest, 8 sets.

2 Mountain climber »

25 seconds work, 45–60 seconds rest, 8 sets.

3 Medicine ball slam/Bodyweight slam »

25 seconds work, 45–60 seconds rest, 8 sets.

DAY OFF

SESSION 3 RESISTANCE LOWER BODY, SUPERSET, TEMPO 4.1.1

1a Barbell front squat/Goblet squat »

10 reps, 90 seconds rest, go straight on to exercise 1b.

1b Walking lunge/Forward lunge »

10 reps, 90 seconds rest, return to exercise 1a. Perform 10 complete sets.

2a Glute bridge/Weighted glute bridge »

10 reps, 60–80 seconds rest, go straight on to exercise 2b.

2b Calf-raise/Machine-assisted calf-raise »

10 reps, 60–80 seconds rest, return to exercise 2a. Perform 6 complete sets.

SESSION 3 HIIT, CIRCUITS

1 Dive-bomber press-up »

25 seconds work, no rest, go straight on to next exercise.

2 Low rotational chop »

25 seconds work, no rest, go straight on to next exercise.

3 Seal jack »

25 seconds work, no rest, go straight on to next exercise.

4 Decline press-up/Normal press-up/Kneeling press-up »

25 seconds work. Rest for 2 minutes post finishing the entire circuit. Perform 4–6 complete circuits.

SESSION 4 RESISTANCE UPPER BODY, SUPERSET, TEMPO 4.1.4

1a Incline dumbbell press/Incline dumbbell fly/Machine press »

10 reps, 90 seconds rest, go straight on exercise 1b.

1b Single-arm dumbbell row/ Cable row/Machine row »

10 reps, 90 seconds rest, return to exercise 1a. Perform 10 complete sets.

2 Barbell upright row/Dumbbell upright row/Kettlebell upright row »

10 reps, 60–80 seconds rest, 6 sets.

3a EZ bar curl/Barbell curl »

10 reps, 60–80 seconds rest, go straight on to exercise 3b.

3b Tricep rope push-down »

10 reps, 60–80 seconds rest, return to exercise 3a. Perform 6 complete sets.

SESSION 4 HIIT, STAND-ALONE EXERCISES

1 Treadmill run/Other cardio equipment run »

25 seconds work, 45–60 seconds rest, 8 sets.

2 Medicine ball slam/Bodyweight slam »

25 seconds work, 45–60 seconds rest, 8 sets.

3 Star jump »

25 seconds work, 45–60 seconds rest, 8 sets.

SESSION 5 RESISTANCE FULL BODY, SUPERSET, TEMPO 4.1.1

1a Bulgarian split squat »

10 reps each side, 60–80 seconds rest, go straight on to exercise 1b.

1b Hamstring extension/Romanian deadlift »

10 reps, 60–80 seconds rest, return to exercise 1a. Perform 5 complete sets.

2a Cable face-pull »

10 reps each side, 60–80 seconds rest, go straight on to exercise 2b.

2b Single-arm dumbbell row/ Cable row/Machine row »

10 reps, 60–80 seconds rest, return to exercise 2a. Perform 4 complete sets.

3a Seated hammer curl »

10 reps each side, 60–80 seconds rest, go straight on to exercise 3b.

3b Close-grip bench press/Narrow hand placement press-up »

10 reps, 60–80 seconds rest, return to exercise 3a. Perform 4 complete sets.

SESSION 5 HIIT, STAND-ALONE EXERCISES

1 Spin bike/Cross-trainer run »

25 seconds work, 45–60 seconds rest, 8 sets.

2 Carioca »

25 seconds work, 45–60 seconds rest, 8 sets.

3 Squat jump »

25 seconds work, 45–60 seconds rest, 8 sets.

DAY OFF

12-WEEK TRAINING PLAN WEEK 6

SESSION 1 RESISTANCE LOWER BODY, SUPERSET, TEMPO 4.1.1

1a Barbell back squat/Dumbbell Squat »

10 reps, 90 seconds rest, go straight on to exercise 1b.

1b Swiss ball hamstring pull/Hamstring curl »

10 reps, 90 seconds rest, return to exercise 1a. Perform 10 complete sets.

2a Deadlift/Trap bar deadlift »

10 reps, 60–80 seconds rest, go straight on to exercise 2b.

2b Calf-raise/Machine-assisted calf-raise »

10 reps, 90 seconds rest, return to exercise 2a. Perform 6 complete sets.

SESSION 1 HIIT, STAND-ALONE EXERCISES

1 Kettlebell swing »

25 seconds work, 45–60 seconds rest, 8 sets.

2 In-and-out squat »

25 seconds work, 45–60 seconds rest, 8 sets.

3 Break dancer »

25 seconds work, 45–60 seconds rest, 8 sets.

SESSION 2 RESISTANCE UPPER BODY, SUPERSET, TEMPO 4.1.1

1a Dumbbell bench press/Dumbbell fly/Machine press »

10 reps, 90 seconds rest, go straight on to exercise 1b.

1b Barbell bent-over row/Seated cable row/Prone row »

10 reps, 90 seconds rest, return to exercise 1a. Perform 10 complete sets.

2 Military press/Shoulder press/Seated shoulder press »

10 reps, 60–80 seconds rest, 6 sets.

3a Chin-up/Counterweight chin-up/Lateral pull-down »

10 reps, go straight on to exercise 3b.

3b Bodyweight dip/Counterweight dip/Tricep rope push-down »

10 reps, 60–80 seconds rest, return to exercise 3a. Perform 6 complete sets.

SESSION 2 HIIT, STAND-ALONE EXERCISES

1 Running on the spot with burpees »

25 seconds work, 45–60 seconds rest, 8 sets.

2 Jumping mountain climber »

25 seconds work, 45–60 seconds rest, 8 sets.

3 Medicine ball slam/Bodyweight slam »

25 seconds work, 45–60 seconds rest, 8 sets.

DAY OFF

SESSION 3 RESISTANCE LOWER BODY, SUPERSET, TEMPO 4.1.1

1a Barbell front squat/Goblet squat »

10 reps, 90 seconds rest, go straight on to exercise 1b.

1b Walking lunge/Forward lunge »

10 reps, 90 seconds rest, return to exercise 1a. Perform 10 complete sets.

2a Glute bridge »

10 reps, 60–80 seconds rest, go straight on to exercise 2b.

2b Calf-raise/Machine-assisted calf-raise »

10 reps, 60–80 seconds rest, return to exercise 2a. Perform 6 complete sets.

SESSION 3 HIIT, CIRCUITS

1 Squat jump »

25 seconds work, no rest, go straight on to next exercise.

2 Press-up/Kneeling press-up »

25 seconds work, no rest, go straight on to next exercise.

3 Lunge change-up/Walking lunge »

25 seconds work, no rest, go straight on to next exercise.

4 Kettlebell standing clean to press »

25 seconds work, rest for 2 minutes post finishing the entire circuit. Perform 4–6 complete circuits.

SESSION 4 RESISTANCE UPPER BODY, SUPERSET, TEMPO 4.1.4

1a Incline dumbbell press/Incline dumbbell fly/Machine press »

10 reps, 90 seconds rest, go straight on to exercise 1b.

1b Single-arm dumbbell row/ Cable row/Machine row »

10 reps, 90 seconds rest, return to exercise 1a. Perform 10 complete sets.

2 Barbell upright row/Kettlebell upright row »

10 reps, 60–80 seconds rest, 6 sets.

3a EZ bar curl/Barbell curl »

10 reps, 60–80 seconds rest, go straight on to exercise 3b.

3b Tricep rope push-down »

10 reps, 60–80 seconds rest, return to exercise 3a. Perform 6 complete sets.

SESSION 4 HIIT, STAND-ALONE EXERCISES

1 Rowing machine/Cardio equipment sprint »

25 seconds work, 45–60 seconds rest, 8 sets.

2 Full body crunch »

25 seconds work, 45–60 seconds rest, 8 sets.

3 Boxing with small dumbbells »

25 seconds work, 45–60 seconds rest, 8 sets.

SESSION 5 RESISTANCE FULL BODY, SUPERSET, TEMPO 4.1.1

1a Bulgarian split squat »

10 reps each side, 60–80 seconds rest, go straight on to exercise 1b.

1b Hamstring extension/Romanian deadlift »

10 reps, 60–80 seconds rest, return to exercise 1a. Perform 5 complete sets.

2a Cable face-pull »

10 reps each side, 60–80 seconds rest, go straight on to exercise 2b.

2b Single-arm dumbbell row/ Cable row/Machine row »

10 reps, 60–80 seconds rest, return to exercise 2a. Perform 4 complete sets.

3a Seated hammer curl »

10 reps each side, 60–80 seconds rest, go straight on to exercise 3b.

3b Close-grip bench press/Narrow hand placement tricep press-up »

10 reps, 60–80 seconds rest, return to exercise 3a. Perform 4 complete sets.

SESSION 5 HIIT, STAND-ALONE EXERCISES

1 Running on the spot »

25 seconds work, 45–60 seconds rest, 8 sets.

2 Straight-leg abdominal flutter »

25 seconds work, 45–60 seconds rest, 8 sets.

3 Full body crunch »

25 seconds work, 45–60 seconds rest, 8 sets.

DAY OFF

We're now into download week, where you are asked to reduce the intensity of your training without actually stopping. The weighted load has been reduced or removed from a lot of the exercises that follow, meaning that you are doing just bodyweight versions. You are also given more days off to allow your body to recover and adapt before things are ramped up again. These alterations will prevent you from plateauing. Please note the following changes:
» The reps, number of sets and tempo have changed, so you should find things a little easier.

SESSION 1 RESISTANCE LOWER BODY, STAND-ALONE EXERCISES, TEMPO 3.1.2

1 Barbell back squat/Dumbbell squat »
6 reps, 60–80 seconds rest, 3 sets.

2 Barbell front squat/Goblet squat »
6 reps, 60–80 seconds rest, 3 sets.

3 Romanian deadlift/Hamstring extension »
6 reps, 60–80 seconds rest, 3 sets.

4 Donkey calf-raise/Machine-assisted calf-raise »
6 reps, 60–80 seconds rest, 6 sets.

SESSION 1 HIIT, CIRCUITS

1 Running on the spot with tuck jumps »
20 seconds work, no rest, go straight on to next exercise.

2 Spiderman mountain climber »
20 seconds work, no rest, go straight on to next exercise.

3 Running off and on a low box »
20 seconds work, no rest, go straight on to next exercise.

4 Side-lying open »
20 seconds work, rest for 2 minutes post finishing the entire circuit. Perform 3–5 complete circuits.

SESSION 2 RESISTANCE UPPER BODY, STAND-ALONE EXERCISES, TEMPO 3.1.2

1 Incline dumbbell fly/Dumbbell fly »
6 reps, 60–80 seconds rest, 3 sets.

2 Incline dumbbell reverse row/Prone row »
6 reps, 60–80 seconds rest, 3 sets.

3 Seated lateral raise »
6 reps, 60–80 seconds rest, 3 sets.

4 Curl to press »
12 reps, 60–80 seconds rest, 3 sets.

5 EZ bar skull-crusher »
12 reps, 60–80 seconds rest, 3 sets.

SESSION 2 HIIT, CIRCUITS

1 Running on the spot with down and ups every 5 seconds »
20 seconds work, 45–60 seconds rest, 4 sets.

2 Kettlebell swing »
20 seconds work, 45–60 seconds rest, 4 sets.

3 Speed walk-out press-up »
20 seconds work, 45–60 seconds rest, 4 sets.

SESSION 3 RESISTANCE LOWER BODY, STAND-ALONE EXERCISES, TEMPO 3.1.2

1 Bulgarian split squat »
6 reps each side, 60–80 seconds rest, 3 sets.

2 Swiss ball hamstring curl/Hamstring curl »
6 reps, 60–80 seconds rest, 3 sets.

3 Calf-raise/Machine-assisted calf-raise »
10 each side, 60–80 seconds rest, 2 sets.

4 Leg press »
10–15 reps, 60–80 seconds rest, 2 sets.

SESSION 3 HIIT, CIRCUITS

1 Side-to-side shuffle »

20 seconds work, no rest, go straight on to next exercise.

2 Lunge change-up/Walking lunge »

20 seconds work, no rest, go straight on to next exercise.

3 Star jump »

20 seconds work, no rest, go straight on to next exercise.

4 Bear crawl »

20 seconds work, no rest, go straight on to next exercise.

5 Boxing while running on the spot »

20 seconds work. Rest for 3 minutes post finishing the entire circuit. Perform 4 complete circuits.

SESSION 4 RESISTANCE UPPER BODY, SUPER SET, TEMPO 3.1.2

1a Decline dumbbell press/Decline press-up »

6 reps, go straight on to exercise 1b.

1b Cable face-pull »

10 reps, 60–80 seconds rest, return to exercise 1a. Perform 3 complete sets.

2a Seated shoulder press/Machine shoulder press »

6 reps, go straight on to exercise 2b.

2b Chin-up/Machine-assisted chin-up/Lateral pull-down »

8 reps, 60–80 seconds rest, return to exercise 2a. Perform 2 complete sets.

3 Prone dumbbell pull-over »

8 reps, 60–80 seconds rest, 2 sets.

SESSION 4 HIIT, STAND-ALONE EXERCISES

1 Broadjump to backward hop »

20 seconds work, 60 seconds rest, 5 sets.

2 Dive-bomber press-up »

20 seconds work, 60 seconds rest, 5 sets.

3 Seal jack »

20 seconds work, 60 seconds rest, 5 sets.

4 Battle ropes »

20 seconds work, 60 seconds rest, 5 sets.

SESSION 5 RESISTANCE FULL BODY, STAND-ALONE EXERCISES, TEMPO 3.1.2

1 Barbell step-up/Dumbbell step-up/Bodyweight step-up »

6 reps each side, 60–80 seconds rest, 3 sets.

2 Weighted glute bridge/Bodyweight glute bridge »

6 reps, 60–80 seconds rest, 3 sets.

3 Press-up/Kneeling press-up »

10 reps, 60–80 seconds rest, 3 sets.

4 Incline reverse lateral raise »

6 reps, 60–80 seconds rest, 2 sets.

5 Barbell bent-over row/Dumbbell bent-over row/Prone row »

6 reps, 60–80 seconds rest, 2 sets.

6 EZ bar reverse curl/Barbell reverse curl/Dumbbell reverse curl »

20–25 reps, 60–80 seconds rest, 2 sets.

SESSION 5 HIIT, STAND-ALONE EXERCISES

1 Mountain climber to burpee (every 5 mountain climbers perform a burpee) »

20 seconds work, 60 seconds rest, 4 sets.

2 Fast feet on the spot »

20 seconds work, 60 seconds rest, 4 sets.

3 Side-to-side hop »

20 seconds work, 60 seconds rest, 4 sets.

4 Front plank with hand tap, done dynamically »

20 seconds work, 60 seconds rest, 4 sets.

DAY OFF

12-WEEK TRAINING PLAN WEEK 8

The idea this week is to build you back up to super-high-intensity training. Please note the following changes:
» The rest times and tempo have changed for some of the exercises.

SESSION 1 RESISTANCE LOWER BODY, SUPERSET, TEMPO 4.1.1

1a Barbell back squat/
Dumbbell squat »

10 reps, 60 seconds rest, go straight on to exercise 1b.

1b Barbell front squat/Goblet squat »

10 reps, 90 seconds rest, return to exercise 1a. Perform 5 complete sets.

2a Barbell Romanian deadlift/
Dumbbell or kettlebell Romanian deadlift »

10 reps, 60 seconds rest, move straight on to exercise 2b.

2b Donkey calf-raise »

20 reps each side, 90 seconds rest, return to exercise 2a. Perform 3 complete sets.

SESSION 1 HIIT, CIRCUITS

1 Bear crawl »

25 seconds work, no rest, go straight on to next exercise.

2 Press-up to break dancer »

25 seconds work, no rest, go straight on to next exercise.

3 Running on the spot with burpees »

25 seconds work, no rest, go straight on to next exercise.

4 Side-lying open »

25 seconds work. Rest for 2 minutes post finishing the entire circuit. Perform 5–8 complete circuits.

SESSION 2 RESISTANCE UPPER BODY, SUPERSET, TEMPO 4.1.1

1a Incline dumbbell fly/Dumbbell fly »

10 reps, 60 seconds rest, move straight on to exercise 1b.

1b Incline dumbbell reverse row/
Prone row »

10 reps, 90 seconds rest, return to exercise 1a. Perform 5 complete sets.

2 Seated lateral raise »

10 reps, 80 seconds rest, 5 sets.

3a Curl to press »

12 reps (6 each side), 60 seconds rest, go straight on to exercise 3b.

3b EZ bar skull-crusher »

12 reps, 80 seconds rest, return to exercise 3a. Perform 3 complete sets.

SESSION 2 HIIT, STAND-ALONE EXERCISES

1 Spin bike/Wattbike/Cross-trainer/
VersaClimber/Cardio equipment run »

25 seconds work, 45–60 seconds rest, 8 sets.

2 Dumbbell thruster »

25 seconds work, 45–60 seconds rest, 8 sets.

3 Lunge change-up »

25 seconds work, 45–60 seconds rest, 8 sets.

SESSION 3 RESISTANCE LOWER BODY, SUPERSET, TEMPO 4.1.1

1a Bulgarian split squat/Bodyweight Bulgarian split squat »

8 reps each side, 60 seconds rest, go straight on to exercise 1b.

1b Swiss ball hamstring pull/
Hamstring curl »

10 reps, 60 seconds rest, return to exercise a. Perform 5 complete sets.

2a Calf-raise/Machine-assisted calf-raise »

20 reps, 60 seconds rest, 3 sets.

2b Leg press »

15–20 reps, 80 seconds rest, 2 sets.

SESSION 3 HIIT, STAND-ALONE EXERCISES

1 Squat jump ››

25 seconds work, 45–60 seconds rest, 8 sets.

2 Burpee/Down and up ››

25 seconds work, 45–60 seconds rest, 8 sets.

3 Side-lying open ››

25 seconds work, 45–60 seconds rest, 8 sets.

4 Seal jack ››

25 seconds work, 45–60 seconds rest, 8 sets.

SESSION 4 RESISTANCE UPPER BODY, SUPERSET, TEMPO 4.1.1

1a Decline dumbbell press/
Decline press-up ››

10 reps, no rest, go straight on to exercise 1b.

1b Cable face-pull ››

10 reps, 60–80 seconds rest, return to exercise 1a. Perform 5 complete sets.

2 Seated shoulder press/
Machine shoulder press ››

10 reps, 60 seconds rest, 5 sets.

3a Neutral-grip chin-up/Machine-assisted neutral-grip chin-up/
Neutral-grip lateral pull-down ››

10 reps, 60 seconds rest, go straight on to exercise 3b.

3b Prone dumbbell pull-over ››

10 reps, 60–80 seconds rest, return to exercise 3a. Perform 3 complete sets.

SESSION 4 HIIT, STAND-ALONE EXERCISES

1 Side-to-side hop ››

25 seconds work, 45–60 seconds rest, 8 sets.

2 Mountain climber ››

25 seconds work, 45–60 seconds rest, 8 sets.

3 Skier swing ››

25 seconds work, 45–60 seconds rest, 8 sets.

4 Front plank with hand tap ››

25 seconds work, 45–60 seconds rest, 8 sets.

SESSION 5 RESISTANCE FULL BODY, STAND-ALONE EXERCISES, TEMPO 4.1.1

1 Barbell step-up/Dumbbell step-up/
Bodyweight step-up ››

8 reps each side, 60–80 seconds rest, 5 sets.

2 Weighted glute bridge/Bodyweight glute bridge ››

10 reps, 60–80 seconds rest, 5 sets.

3 Press-up/Kneeling press-up ››

10 reps, 60–80 seconds rest, 3 sets.

4 Incline reverse lateral raise ››

8 reps, 60–80 seconds rest, 3 sets.

5 Barbell bent-over row/Dumbbell bent-over row/Prone row ››

8 reps, 60–80 seconds rest, 3 sets.

6 EZ bar reverse curl/Barbell reverse curl/Dumbbell reverse curl ››

20–25 reps, 60–80 seconds rest, 2 sets.

SESSION 5 HIIT, CIRCUITS

1 Running on the spot with high knees ››

25 seconds work, no rest, go straight on to next exercise.

2 Bodyweight squat ››

25 seconds work, no rest, go straight on to next exercise.

3 Press-up to burpee ››

25 seconds work, no rest, go straight on to next exercise.

4 Jumping mountain climber ››

25 seconds work, rest for 2 minutes post finishing the entire circuit. Perform 4–6 complete circuits.

DAY OFF

We're now fully back into high-intensity training. Please note the following changes:
>> The work time has increased from 25 seconds to 30.
>> Rest times have changed for certain exercises.
>> Tempo is now 4.0.1.
>> Each workout has 10 sets of 10.
>> An extra exercise has been added to some HIIT sessions.

SESSION 1 RESISTANCE LOWER BODY, SUPERSET, TEMPO 4.0.1

1a Barbell back squat/Dumbbell squat »

10 reps, 90 seconds rest, go straight on to exercise 1b.

1b Barbell front squat/Goblet squat »

10 reps, 90 seconds rest, return to exercise 1a. Perform 10 complete sets.

2a Romanian deadlift/Dumbbell or kettlebell Romanian deadlift »

10 reps, 90 seconds rest, go straight on to exercise 2b.

2b Donkey calf-raise »

20 reps each side, rest 90 seconds, return to exercise. Perform 6 complete sets.

SESSION 1 HIIT, CIRCUITS

1 Skipping on the spot with a rope/ Skipping on the spot without a rope »

30 seconds work, 60 seconds rest, 8 sets.

2 Side-to-side hop »

30 seconds work, 60 seconds rest, 8 sets.

3 Speed walk-out press-up »

30 seconds work, 60 seconds rest, 8 sets.

SESSION 2 RESISTANCE UPPER BODY, SUPERSET, TEMPO 4.0.1

1a Incline dumbbell fly/Dumbbell fly »

10 reps, 90 seconds rest, go straight on to exercise 1b.

1b Incline dumbbell reverse row/ Prone row »

10 reps, 90 seconds rest, return to exercise 1a. Perform 10 complete sets.

2 Seated lateral raise »

10 reps, 90 seconds rest, 10 sets.

3a Curl to press »

12 reps (6 each side), 60 seconds rest, go straight on to exercise 3b.

3b EZ bar skull-crusher »

12 reps, 80 seconds rest, return to exercise 3a. Perform 6 complete sets.

SESSION 2 HIIT, CIRCUITS

1 Treadmill run/Other cardio equipment run »

30 seconds work, no rest, go straight on to next exercise.

2 Burpee/Down and up »

30 seconds work, no rest, go straight on to next exercise.

3 Dive-bomber press-up/Normal press up »

30 seconds work, no rest, go straight on to next exercise.

4 Diagonal rotational chop »

30 seconds work, rest for 2 minutes post finishing the entire circuit. Perform 5–8 complete circuits.

SESSION 3 RESISTANCE LOWER BODY, SUPERSET, TEMPO 4.0.1

1a Bulgarian split squat/Bodyweight Bulgarian split squat »

10 reps each side, 90 seconds rest, go straight on to exercise 1b.

1b Swiss ball hamstring pull/Hamstring curl »

10 reps, 90 seconds rest, return to exercise 1a. Perform 10 complete sets.

2 Calf-raise/Machine-assisted calf-raise »

20 reps, 60 seconds rest, perform 6 complete sets, go straight on to exercise 2b.

3 Leg press »

15–20 reps, 80 seconds rest. Perform 3 complete sets.

SESSION 3 HIIT, CIRCUITS

1 Boxing forwards and upwards while running on the spot »

30 seconds work, no rest, go straight on to next exercise.

2 Mountain climber to burpee (every 5 seconds perform a burpee) »

30 seconds work, no rest, go straight on to next exercise.

3 Seal jack »

30 seconds work, no rest, go straight on to next exercise.

4 Side-lying open »

30 seconds work, rest for 2 minutes post finishing the entire circuit. Perform 5–8 complete circuits.

SESSION 4 RESISTANCE UPPER BODY, SUPERSET, TEMPO 4.0.1

1a Decline dumbbell press/Decline press-up/Normal press-up »

10 reps, no rest, go straight on to exercise 1b.

1b Cable face-pull »

10 reps, 90 seconds rest, return to exercise 1a. Perform 10 complete sets.

2 Seated shoulder press/Machine shoulder press »

10 reps, 60 seconds rest, 10 sets.

3a Neutral-grip chin-up/Counterweight neutral-grip chin-up/Neutral-grip lateral pull-down »

10 reps, 90 seconds rest, go straight on to exercise 3b.

3b Prone dumbbell pull-over »

10 reps, 60–80 seconds rest, return to exercise 3a. Perform 6 complete sets.

SESSION 4 HIIT, STAND-ALONE EXERCISES

1 Running on the spot with butt kicks »

30 seconds work, 45–60 seconds rest, 8 sets.

2 Skater jump »

30 seconds work, 45–60 seconds rest, 8 sets.

3 Speed walk-out press-up »

30 seconds work, 45–60 seconds rest, 8 sets.

4 Tuck jump »

30 seconds work, 45–60 seconds rest, 8 sets.

SESSION 5 RESISTANCE FULL BODY, STAND-ALONE EXERCISES, TEMPO 4.0.1

1 Barbell step-up/Dumbbell step-up/Bodyweight step-up »

8 reps each side, 60–80 seconds rest, 6 sets.

2 Weighted glute bridge/Bodyweight glute bridge »

10 reps, 60–80 seconds rest, 6 sets.

3 Press-up/Kneeling press-up »

10 reps, 60–80 seconds rest, 6 sets.

4 Incline reverse lateral raise »

8 reps, 60–80 seconds rest, 4 sets.

5 Barbell bent-over row/Dumbbell bent-over row/Prone row »

8 reps, 60–80 seconds rest, 4 sets.

6 EZ bar reverse curl/Barbell reverse curl/Dumbbell reverse curl »

20–25 reps, 60–80 seconds rest, 2 sets.

SESSION 5 HIIT, STAND-ALONE EXERCISES

1 Boxing forwards and upwards while running on the spot »

25 seconds work, 45–60 seconds rest, 8 sets.

2 Carioca »

25 seconds work, 45–60 seconds rest, 8 sets.

3 Squat jump »

25 seconds work, 45–60 seconds rest, 8 sets.

4 Seal jack »

25 seconds work, 45–60 seconds rest, 8 sets.

DAY OFF

Please note the following changes:
>> The number of reps has altered.
>> You are still doing 10 sets of some exercises, but are dropping to only 6 reps.

SESSION 1 RESISTANCE LOWER BODY, SUPERSET, TEMPO 4.0.1

1a Barbell back squat/Dumbbell squat »

6 reps, 90 seconds rest, go straight on to exercise 1b.

1b Front squat/Goblet squat »

6 reps, 90 seconds rest, return to exercise 1a. Perform 10 complete sets.

2a Romanian deadlift/Dumbbell or kettlebell Romanian deadlift »

10 reps, 90 seconds rest, go straight on to exercise 2b.

2b Donkey calf-raise »

20 reps each side, 90 seconds rest, return to exercise 2a. Perform 5 complete sets.

SESSION 1 HIIT, CIRCUITS

1 Side-to-side shuffle »

30 seconds work, no rest, go straight on to next exercise.

2 Diagonal rotational chop »

30 seconds work, no rest, go straight on to next exercise.

3 Decline press-up/Normal press-up »

30 seconds work, rest for 2 minutes post finishing the entire circuit. Perform 4–6 complete circuits.

SESSION 2 RESISTANCE UPPER BODY, SUPERSET, TEMPO 4.0.1

1a Incline dumbbell fly/Dumbbell fly »

6 reps, 90 seconds rest, go straight on to exercise 1b.

1b Incline dumbbell reverse row/Prone row »

6 reps, 90 seconds rest, return to exercise 1a. Perform 10 complete sets.

2 Seated lateral raise »

6 reps, 90 seconds rest, 10 sets.

3a Curl to press »

12 reps (6 each side), 60 seconds rest, go straight on to exercise 3b.

3b EZ bar skull-crusher »

12 reps, 80 seconds rest, return to exercise 3a. Perform 5 complete sets.

SESSION 2 HIIT, STAND-ALONE EXERCISES

1 Treadmill run/Other cardio equipment sprint »

30 seconds work, 45–60 seconds rest, 8 sets.

2 Drop squat »

30 seconds work, 45–60 seconds rest, 8 sets.

3 Medicine ball slam »

30 seconds work, 45–60 seconds rest, 8 sets.

4 Speed walk-out press-up »

30 seconds work, 8 sets.

SESSION 3 RESISTANCE LOWER BODY, SUPERSET, TEMPO 4.1.1

1a Bulgarian split squat/Bodyweight Bulgarian split squat »

6 reps each side, 90 seconds rest, go straight on to exercise 1b.

1b Swiss ball hamstring pull/Hamstring curl »

6 reps, 90 seconds rest, return to exercise 1a. Perform 10 complete sets.

2a Calf-raise »

20 reps, 60 seconds rest, 5 sets.

2b Leg press »

15–20 reps, 90 seconds rest, 3 sets.

SESSION 3 HIIT, STAND-ALONE EXERCISES

1 Running on the spot with tuck jumps »

30 seconds work, 45–60 seconds rest, 8 sets.

2 Carioca side-to-side »

30 seconds work, 45–60 seconds rest, 8 sets.

3 Squat jump »

30 seconds work, 45–60 seconds rest, 8 sets.

4 Dive bomber press-ups »

30 seconds work, 45–60 seconds rest, 8 sets.

SESSION 4 RESISTANCE UPPER BODY, SUPERSET, TEMPO 4.1.1

1a Decline dumbbell press/Decline press-up/Normal press-up »

6 reps, no rest, go straight on to exercise 1b.

1b Cable face-pull »

6 reps, 90 seconds rest, return to exercise 1a. Perform 10 complete sets.

2 Seated shoulder press/Machine shoulder press »

6 reps, 60 seconds rest, 10 sets.

3a Chin-up/Counterweight chin-up/Lateral pull-down »

10 reps, 90 seconds rest, go straight on to exercise 3b.

3b Prone dumbbell pull-over »

10 reps, 60–80 seconds rest, return to exercise 3a. Perform 4 complete sets.

SESSION 4 HIIT, STAND-ALONE EXERCISES

1 Skipping on the spot with a rope/Skipping on the spot without a rope »

30 seconds work, 45–60 seconds rest, 8 sets.

2 Drop squat »

30 seconds work, 45–60 seconds rest, 8 sets.

3 Mountain climber to burpee (every 5 seconds perform a burpee) »

30 seconds work, 45–60 seconds rest, 8 sets.

4 Side-lying open »

30 seconds work, 45–60 seconds rest, 8 sets.

SESSION 5 RESISTANCE FULL BODY, STAND-ALONE EXERCISES, TEMPO 4.1.1

1 Barbell step-up/Dumbbell step-up/Bodyweight step-up »

8 reps each side, 60–80 seconds rest, 6 sets.

2 Weighted glute bridge/Bodyweight glute bridge »

10 reps, 60–80 seconds rest, 6 sets.

3 Press-up/Kneeling press-up/Wall press-up »

10 reps, 60–80 seconds rest, 6 sets.

4 Incline reverse lateral raise »

8 reps, 60–80 seconds rest, 4 sets.

5 Barbell bent-over row/Dumbbell bent-over row/Prone row »

8 reps, 60–80 seconds rest, 4 sets.

6 EZ bar reverse curl/Barbell reverse curl/Dumbbell reverse curl »

20–25 reps, 60–80 seconds rest, 2 sets.

SESSION 5 HIIT, STAND-ALONE EXERCISES

1 Bear crawl »

30 seconds work, 45–60 seconds rest, 8 sets.

2 Carioca »

30 seconds work, 45–60 seconds rest, 8 sets.

3 Medicine ball slam/Bodyweight slam »

30 seconds work, 45–60 seconds rest, 8 sets.

4 Front plank with hand tap »

30 seconds work, 45–60 seconds rest, 8 sets.

DAY OFF

12-WEEK TRAINING PLAN WEEK 11

SESSION 1 RESISTANCE LOWER BODY, SUPERSET, TEMPO 4.0.1

1a Barbell back squat/Dumbbell squat »

6 reps, 90 seconds rest, go straight on to exercise 1b.

1b Barbell front squat/Goblet squat »

6 reps, 90 seconds rest, return to exercise 1a. Perform 10 complete sets.

2a Romanian deadlift/Dumbbell or kettlebell Romanian deadlift »

10 reps, 90 seconds rest, go straight on to exercise 2b.

2b Donkey calf-raise »

20 reps each side, 90 seconds rest, return to exercise 2a. Perform 5 complete sets.

SESSION 1 HIIT, CIRCUITS

1 Treadmill run/Other cardio equipment run »

30 seconds work, 45–60 seconds rest, 8 sets.

2 Medicine ball slam/Halo slam »

30 seconds work, 45–60 seconds rest, 8 sets.

3 Drop squat »

30 seconds work, 45–60 seconds rest, 8 sets.

4 Star jump »

30 seconds work, 45–60 seconds rest, 8 sets. Rest for 2 minutes post finishing the entire circuit. Perform 5–8 complete circuits.

SESSION 2 RESISTANCE UPPER BODY, SUPERSET, TEMPO 4.0.1

1a Incline dumbbell fly/Dumbbell fly »

6 reps, 90 seconds rest, move straight on to exercise 1b.

1b Incline dumbbell reverse row »

6 reps, 90 seconds rest, return to exercise 1a. Perform 10 complete sets.

2 Seated lateral raise »

6 reps, 90 seconds rest, 10 sets.

3a Curl to press »

12 reps (6 each side), 60 seconds rest, go straight on to exercise 3b.

3b EZ bar skull-crusher »

12 reps, 80 seconds rest, return to exercise 3a. Perform 5 complete sets.

SESSION 2 HIIT, STAND-ALONE EXERCISES

1 Running on the spot with tuck jumps »

30 seconds work, 45–60 seconds rest, 8 sets.

2 Spiderman mountain climbers »

30 seconds work, 45–60 seconds rest, 8 sets.

3 Skater jump »

30 seconds work, 45–60 seconds rest, 8 sets.

4 Backwards and forward shuttle »

30 seconds work, 45–60 seconds rest, 8 sets.

SESSION 3 RESISTANCE LOWER BODY, SUPERSET, TEMPO 4.1.1

1a Bulgarian split squat/Bodyweight Bulgarian split squat »

6 reps each side, 90 seconds rest, go straight on to exercise 1b.

1b Swiss ball hamstring pull/Hamstring curl »

6 reps, 90 seconds rest, return to exercise 1a. Perform 10 complete sets.

2 Calf-raise/Machine-assisted calf-raise »

20 reps, 60 seconds rest, 5 sets.

3 Leg press »

15–20 reps, 90 seconds rest, 3 sets.

SESSION 3 HIIT, STAND-ALONE EXERCISES

1 Running on the spot with high knees »

30 seconds work, 45–60 seconds rest, 8 sets.

2 Drop squat »

30 seconds work, 45–60 seconds rest, 8 sets.

3 Dive-bomber press-up »

30 seconds work, 45–60 seconds rest, 8 sets.

4 Broad jump to backward hop »

30 seconds work, 45–60 seconds rest, 8 sets.

SESSION 4 RESISTANCE UPPER BODY, SUPERSET, TEMPO 4.1.1

1a Decline dumbbell press/Decline press-up »

6 reps, go straight on to exercise 1b.

1b Cable face-pull »

6 reps, 90 seconds rest, return to exercise 1a. Perform 10 complete sets.

2 Seated shoulder press/Machine shoulder press »

6 reps, 60 seconds rest, 10 sets.

3a Neutral-grip chin-up/ Counterweight neutral-grip chin-up/ Neutral-grip lateral pull-down »

10 reps, 90 seconds rest, move straight on to exercise 3b.

3b Prone dumbbell pull-over »

10 reps, 60–80 seconds rest, return to exercise 3a. Perform 4 complete sets.

SESSION 4 HIIT, CIRCUITS

1 Fast feet on the spot »

30 seconds work, no rest, go straight on to next exercise.

2 Low rotational chop »

30 seconds work, no rest, go straight on to next exercise.

3 Press-up to break dancer »

30 seconds work, no rest, go straight on to next exercise.

4 Straight-leg abdominal flutter »

25 seconds work. Rest for 2 minutes post finishing the entire circuit. Perform 5–8 complete circuits.

SESSION 5 RESISTANCE FULL BODY, STAND-ALONE EXERCISES, TEMPO 4.1.1

1 Barbell step-up/Dumbbell step-up/ Bodyweight step-up »

8 reps each side, 60–80 seconds rest, 6 sets.

2 Weighted glute bridge/Bodyweight glute bridge »

10 reps, 60–80 seconds rest, 6 sets.

3 Press-up/Kneeling press-up »

10 reps, 60–80 seconds rest, 6 sets.

4 Incline reverse lateral raise »

8 reps, 60–80 seconds rest, 4 sets.

5 Barbell bent-over row/Dumbbell bent-over row/Prone row »

8 reps, 60–80 seconds rest, 4 sets.

6 EZ bar reverse curl/Barbell reverse curl/Dumbbell reverse curl »

20–25 reps, 60–80 seconds rest, 2 sets.

SESSION 5 HIIT, STAND-ALONE EXERCISES

1 Kettlebell swing »

30 seconds work, 45–60 seconds rest, 8 sets.

2 Battle ropes »

30 seconds work, 45–60 seconds rest, 8 sets.

3 Press-up to break dancer »

30 seconds work, 45–60 seconds rest, 8 sets.

4 Medicine ball slam »

30 seconds work, 45–60 seconds rest, 8 sets.

DAY OFF

12-WEEK TRAINING PLAN WEEK 12

Congratulations! You are into your last week of the 12-week programme.

SESSION 1 RESISTANCE LOWER BODY, SUPERSET, TEMPO 4.0.1

1a Barbell back squat/Dumbbell squat »

6 reps, 90 seconds rest, go straight on to exercise 1b.

1b Barbell front squat/Goblet squat »

6 reps, 90 seconds rest, return to exercise 1a. Perform 10 complete sets.

2a Romanian deadlift/Dumbbell or kettlebell Romanian deadlift »

10 reps, 90 seconds rest, move straight on to exercise 2b.

2b Donkey calf-raise »

20 reps each side, 90 seconds rest, return to exercise 2a. Perform 5 complete sets.

SESSION 1 HIIT, STAND-ALONE EXERCISES

1 Spin bike/Cross-trainer run/ Other cardio equipment run »

30 seconds work, 45–60 seconds rest, 8 sets.

2 Carioca »

30 seconds work, 45–60 seconds rest, 8 sets.

3 Fast feet »

30 seconds work, 45–60 seconds rest, 8 sets.

4 Full body crunch »

30 seconds work, 45–60 seconds rest, 8 sets.

SESSION 2 RESISTANCE UPPER BODY, SUPERSET, TEMPO 4.0.1

1a Incline dumbbell fly/Dumbbell fly »

6 reps, 90 seconds rest, go straight on to exercise 1b.

1b Incline dumbbell reverse row »

6 reps, 90 seconds rest, return to exercise 1a. Perform 10 complete sets.

2 Seated lateral raise »

6 reps, 90 seconds rest, 10 sets.

3a Curl to press »

12 reps (6 each side), 60 seconds rest, go straight on to exercise 3b.

3b EZ bar skull-crusher »

12 reps, 80 seconds rest, return to exercise 3a. Perform 5 complete sets.

SESSION 2 HIIT, STAND-ALONE EXERCISES

1 Treadmill run/Other cardio equipment run »

30 seconds work, 45–60 seconds rest, 8 sets.

2 Medicine ball slam/Bodyweight slam »

30 seconds work, 45–60 seconds rest, 8 sets.

3 Jumping mountain climber »

30 seconds work, 45–60 seconds rest, 8 sets.

4 Diagonal rotational chop »

30 seconds work, 45–60 seconds rest, 8 sets.

SESSION 3 RESISTANCE LOWER BODY, SUPERSET, TEMPO 4.1.1

1a Bulgarian split squat/Bodyweight Bulgarian split squat »

6 reps each side, 90 seconds rest, go straight on to exercise 1b.

1b Swiss ball hamstring pull/ Hamstring curl »

6 reps, 90 seconds rest, return to exercise 1a. Perform 10 complete sets.

2 Calf-raise/Machine-assisted calf-raise »

20 reps, 60 seconds rest, 5 sets.

3 Leg press »

15–20 reps, 90 seconds rest, 3 sets.

SESSION 3 HIIT, CIRCUITS

1 Drop squat »

30 seconds work, no rest, go straight on to next exercise.

2 Bear crawl »

30 seconds work, no rest, go straight on to next exercise.

3 Backward and forward shuttle »

30 seconds work, no rest, go straight on to next exercise.

4 Kettlebell standing clean to press »

30 seconds work. Rest for 2 minutes post finishing the entire circuit. Perform 5–8 complete circuits.

SESSION 4 RESISTANCE UPPER BODY, SUPERSET, TEMPO 4.1.1

1a Decline dumbbell press/Decline press-up »

6 reps, go straight on to exercise 2b.

1b Cable face-pull »

6 reps, 90 seconds rest, return to exercise 1a. Perform 10 complete sets.

2 Seated shoulder press/Machine shoulder press »

6 reps, 60 seconds rest, 10 sets.

3a Neutral-grip chin-up/ Counterweight neutral-grip chin-up/ Neutral-grip lateral pull-down »

10 reps, 90 seconds rest, move straight on to exercise 3b.

3b Prone dumbbell pull-over »

10 reps, 60–80 seconds rest, return to exercise 3a. Perform 4 complete sets.

SESSION 4 HIIT, STAND-ALONE EXERCISES

1 Broad jump to backward hop »

30 seconds work, 45–60 seconds rest, 8 sets.

2 Side-to-side hop »

30 seconds work, 45–60 seconds rest, 8 sets.

3 Side plank hold »

30 seconds work, 45–60 seconds rest, 8 sets.

4 Speed walk-out to press-up »

30 seconds work, 45–60 seconds rest, 8 sets.

12-WEEK TRAINING PLAN WEEK 12

SESSION 5 RESISTANCE FULL BODY, STAND-ALONE EXERCISES, TEMPO 4.1.1

1 Barbell step-up/Dumbbell step-up/ Bodyweight step-up »

8 reps each side, 60–80 seconds rest, 6 sets.

2 Weighted glute bridge/Bodyweight glute bridge »

10 reps, 60–80 seconds rest, 6 sets.

3 Press-up/Kneeling press-up »

10 reps, 60–80 seconds rest, 6 sets.

4 Incline reverse lateral raise »

8 reps, 60–80 seconds rest, 4 sets.

5 Barbell bent-over row/Dumbbell bent-over row/Prone row »

8 reps, 60–80 seconds rest, 4 sets.

6 EZ bar reverse curl/Barbell reverse curl/Dumbbell reverse curl »

20–25 reps, 60–80 seconds rest, 2 sets.

SESSION 5 HIIT, STAND-ALONE EXERCISES

1 Kettlebell swing »

30 seconds work, 45–60 seconds rest, 8 sets.

2 Spiderman mountain climbers »

30 seconds work, 45–60 seconds rest, 8 sets.

3 Straight-leg abdominal flutter »

30 seconds work, 45–60 seconds rest, 8 sets.

4 Front plank with hand tap »

30 seconds work, 45–60 seconds rest, 8 sets.

DAY OFF

Congratulations! You have now finished the 12-week plan. You should feel immensely proud of what you have achieved because the plan is not easy and you have worked extremely hard to get through it. You should now have some amazing results and be pleased with what you see in the mirror. If you feel like sharing your progress with me, and the rest of the world, then please do so on any of my social media links:

Twitter: @jameshaskell

Instagram: @jameshask

Facebook: jameshaskelljhhf

If you are wondering what to do next, my advice would be to take a download week or a complete week off, and then start the programme again. This time, with all the knowledge and experience you have gained, you can push yourself even harder.

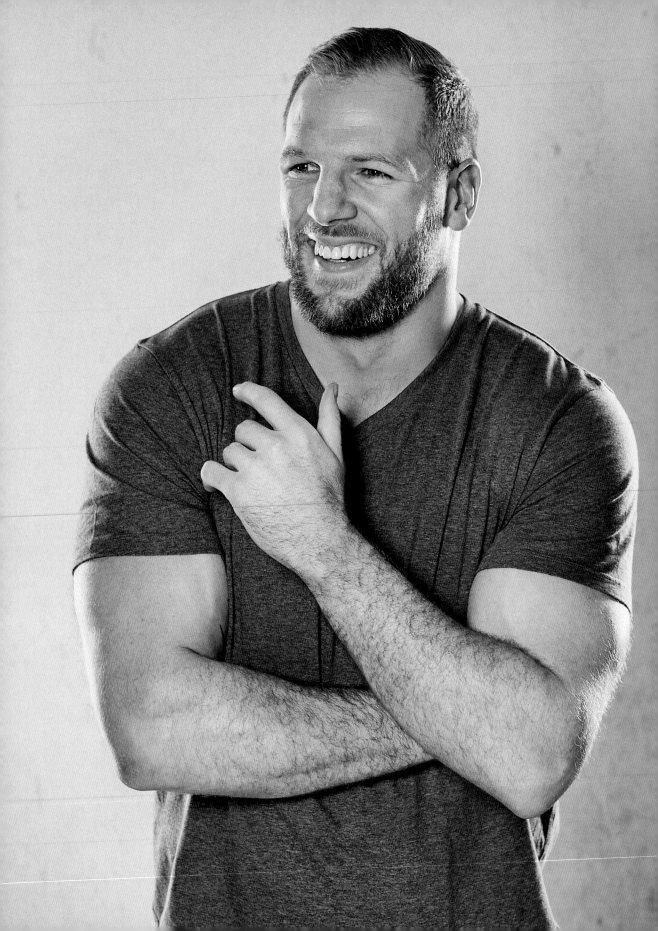

Chapter 4
THE EXERCISES STEP-BY-STEP

All the exercises used in the warm-ups, training sessions and recovery periods can be found in this chapter. For ease of reference, they are arranged in alphabetical order.

It's important to remember that whenever you see more than one exercise suggested in the training plans, I want you ideally to do the first one. The other options are for those who don't have access to the required equipment, or who don't yet have the technique to do it, or who want to start with bodyweight exercises (i.e. without equipment) first.

Remember that most exercises associated with weight training are ideally done weighted unless an alternative is given. For example, Bulgarian split squats are always weighted, but you can do bodyweight Bulgarian split squats where this alternative is given too.

Please read the text as well as looking at the photos to ensure you do everything correctly.

BACK ROLL-OUT

» Lie on the floor and roll yourself into a ball, hugging your knees.

» Slowly roll backwards and forwards, trying to roll out the entirety of your spine.
It's normal for your back to make a few clicks while doing this.

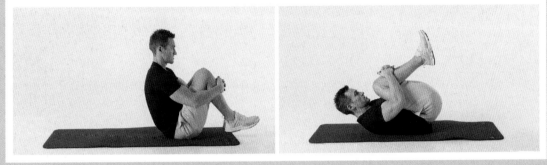

BACKWARD AND FORWARD SHUTTLE

» Decide how far you want to run for this drill and place a marker at either end of the course.
While you will be limited by the space where you are doing the exercise, the cones should
be spaced at least 10 metres apart.

» Run between the two points in a straight line as quickly as you can. The fitter you are,
the more shuttles back and forth you can do in the allotted time.

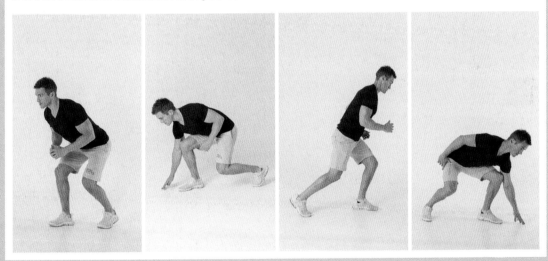

BARBELL BACK SQUAT

» Stand with your feet shoulder width apart.

» Rest a barbell on your traps with a weight you can squat confidently and with perfect form. Grasp the barbell with your hands.

» Making sure you have all your weight in your heels, bend at the knees and drop your bottom towards the floor. Stop at the point when you can no longer maintain perfect form.

» Keep your back straight and make sure your knees drive outwards, rather than buckling inwards.

» At the bottom of the squat, squeeze the bar and drive upwards, keeping your back straight and knees out at all times. Use your hamstrings, glutes and hips to drive you back up.

» Hold your breath as you lower the weight, and exhale near the top of the lift on the way back up. This will keep your abs and back set.

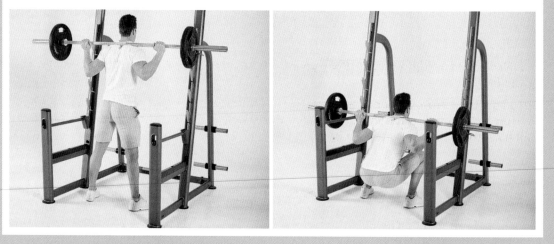

BARBELL BENT-OVER ROW

» Adopt an athletic position with your knees slightly bent. Pick a barbell up from the floor with an overhand grip.

» Bend at the knees until you are just above horizontal, keeping your back flat and your weight in your heels.

» Keeping your back straight, row the weight towards your chest just below your sternum. Focus on squeezing your shoulder blades together as you do this to engage your back muscles.

» Lower the bar with control to the starting position.

» Make sure you keep your head neutral when doing a bent-over row. Too many people arch their neck. Find a spot on the floor just in front of you and focus on it while you lift.

See pictures opposite » » »

»»» Barbell bent-over row

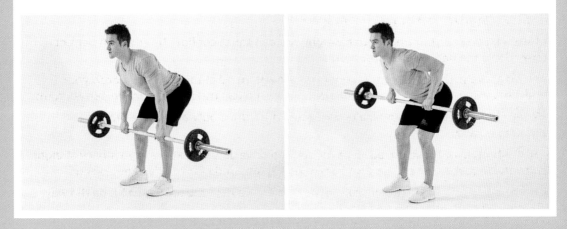

BARBELL CURL

» While standing, hold a barbell. Keep your back straight and feet firmly planted on the ground.

» Curl the bar towards tyour chest, creating maximum tension in your biceps. Ensure you perform a full range of motion and squeeze the muscle at the top of the movement. Do not hoist the weight up with your back.

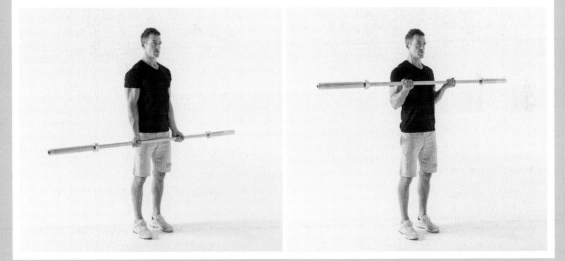

BARBELL FRONT SQUAT

» Stand inside a squat rack with a barbell in front of you at chest height. Rest the barbell at the top of your sternum, pushing it into your neck. You can grip the bar with your wrists bent backwards, or with your arms crossed over the bar. Most people find the second of these options to be the most comfortable.

» Stand with feet, slightly wider than shoulder width apart, back straight and abdominals braced. Drop your bottom towards the floor in a squat, ensuring your knees do not buckle inwards and that your weight is in your heels.

» At the bottom of the squat position, drive your body upwards to return to standing, bracing your abs as you do so.

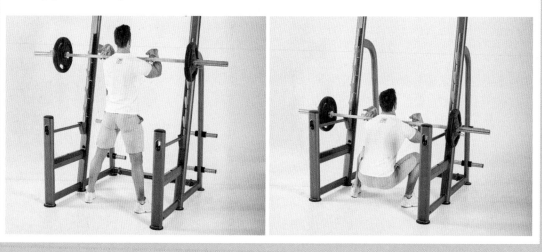

BARBELL REVERSE CURL

» Hold a barbell in front of you, with your palms facing you.

» Curl the bar upwards, but do not turn your wrists. At the top of the movement your palms should be facing away. You should feel the tension in your forearms.

» Lower the weight with control and repeat.

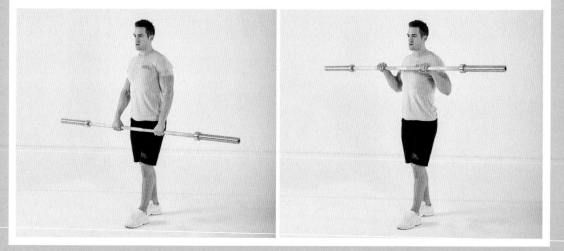

BARBELL STEP-UP

» Stand with your feet shoulder width apart, facing a bench or box set to a height just above your knees.

» Hold a barbell in your hands with an overhand grip.

» Using your left leg, step onto the bench, then follow with your right leg so that both feet are planted on the bench. You can drive your free knee through so that you finish at the top of the movement with both legs on top of the box.

» Lower the left leg to the floor, then follow with your right leg so that both feet are now back on the ground. Make sure you engage your glutes on the way down.

» Repeat the process, this time leading with your right leg.

» To make this exercise harder you can increase the height of the bench or box, and add more weight to the bar. If you don't feel confident enough to do this, just keep working with your bodyweight.

» Always focus on engaging your glutes, or bottom muscles, as you power up and lower down. You should always have tension in this area.

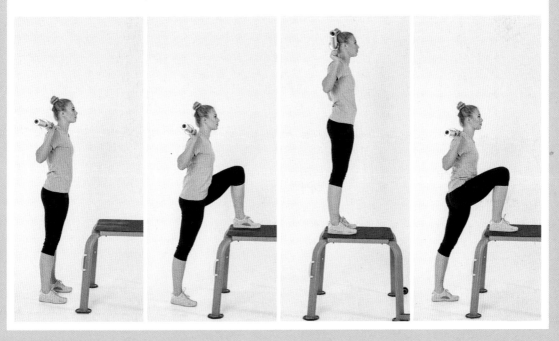

BARBELL UPRIGHT ROW

» Grasp your barbell with an overhand grip and hold it in front of your thighs, arms straight. Your grip should be roughly shoulder width apart.

» Keeping your back straight at all times, raise your elbows up and to the side to lift the weight to the top of your chest. Keep the bar close to your body as you raise it. You should feel this movement in your upper back and traps. If necessary, you can put one foot in front of the other to balance yourself.

» Lower the weight with control to the starting position.

» Do not do half-reps on this exercise. Control the barbell all the way from bottom to top, making sure your elbows travel up first.

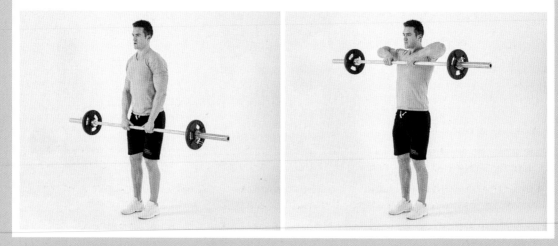

BATTLE ROPES

» Secure a battle rope to a fixed pole, or around a heavy piece of equipment grabbing hold of both ends.

» Lower yourself into a half squat with your back straight, then move your arms up and down to whip the ropes as hard as you can for the specified work time. You can alternate between single-arm whips and double-arm whips.

» Make sure your arms stay close to your body, and that they, rather than your shoulders or whole upper body, do the work.

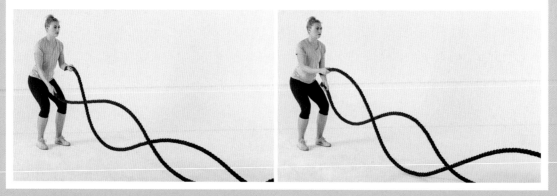

BEAR CRAWL

» Get on all fours like a bear. Your weight is on your hands and toes, with your knees underneath you and off the ground.

» Keeping your back flat, crawl forward rapidly for 10 steps, then reverse for 10 steps. Maintain abdominal tension as you do so.

» Do not allow your back to round or your bottom to come up as you do this exercise.

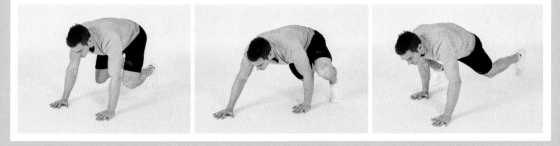

BENCH PRESS

» Lie down on a flat bench under a bench press platform. Grasp the bar at shoulder width or slightly wider and hold it above your head with your arms fully extended.

» Lower the bar with control until it is 1–2cm above your chest. Now drive the bar upwards until your arms are fully extended to the starting position.

» To perform a close grip bench press repeat the action above, with your hands a fist-width apart.

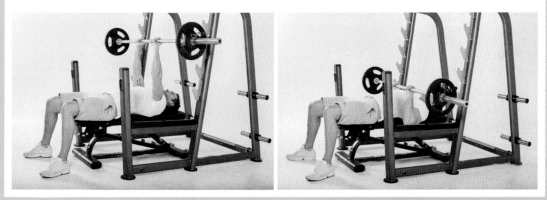

BODYWEIGHT BENCH DIP

» Sit on the edge of a bench, placing your hands behind you so that they are resting on the bench. They should be about shoulder width apart with elbows straight.

» Stretch out your legs so that they are at a 90° angle, using your hands to support your bodyweight. Now bend at the elbow and lower your body with control until your arms are at a 90° angle.

» Push yourself back up to straighten your arms, contracting your triceps as you do so. Repeat as necessary.

» To make this movement harder you can stretch your legs so they are straight or rest your feet on an elevated surface to increase the range of motion.

» If you want to develop big arms, triceps are key, so make sure you go through the full range of movement.

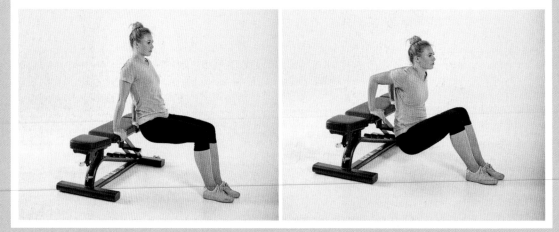

BODYWEIGHT DIP

» Hold your bodyweight above two dipping bars at approximately shoulder width apart or just wider. Your arms should be straight and your abdominals engaged.

» Lower your body with control between the dipping bars until your elbows are at right angles and your chest is level with the bars. Now explode back up to the starting position, engaging your triceps and chest as you do so.

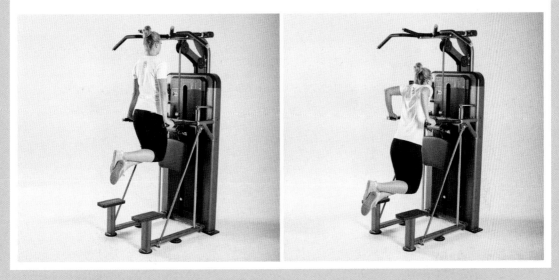

BODYWEIGHT SLAM

» Start with your feet shoulder width apart and adopt an athletic position, knees slightly bent.

» Clasp your hands together in a tight grip – fingers interlocked works best – and rest them in front of you, arms straight.

» Lift your arms above your head, keeping your abs and glutes engaged. As you do this, your knees should straighten.

» When your arms are fully extended, brace your core, bend at the knees and slam your arms down to the starting position. You should maintain full abdominal tension throughout this movement.

» Don't allow your back to start curling when you do this exercise. Slam down and then come back to standing.

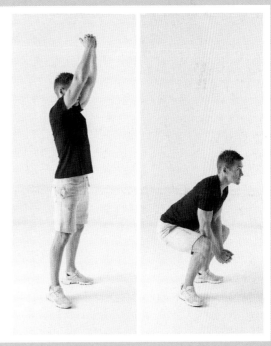

BODYWEIGHT SQUAT

» Always think about keeping your weight through your heels and your knees tracking out when you squat.

» Stand with your feet shoulder width apart, keeping all your weight on your heels.

» Drop your bottom towards the floor, adopting a squat position while keeping your abs tight and your back straight.

» Do not allow your knees to buckle inwards. You must keep them out and tracking over your feet.

» Using your hamstrings, glutes and hips, drive back up to your starting position. Unless stated otherwise, the raising phase is more dynamic that the lowering phase.

» Squat only as deep as you can while maintaining good form. If you can't keep your back flat, or your weight through your heels, or your spine from curving, reduce the depth of your squat until you have excellent form.

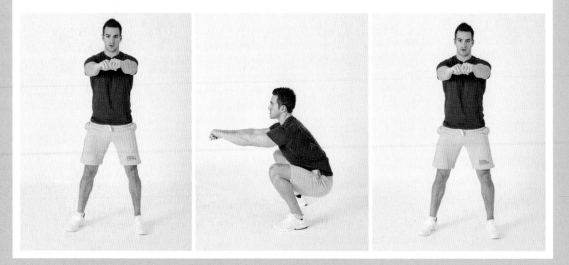

BODYWEIGHT STEP-UP

» Stand with your feet shoulder width apart facing a bench or box set to a height just above knee level. Step onto with your left leg, then follow with your right leg so that both feet are planted on the bench.

» Take your left leg back to the floor, then follow with your right leg so that both feet are now back on the ground.

» Repeat this process, leading first with your right leg.

» To make this exercise harder you can increase the height of the bench or box, or add resistance in the form of a barbell or dumbbells.

See pictures opposite »»»

»»» Bodyweight step-up

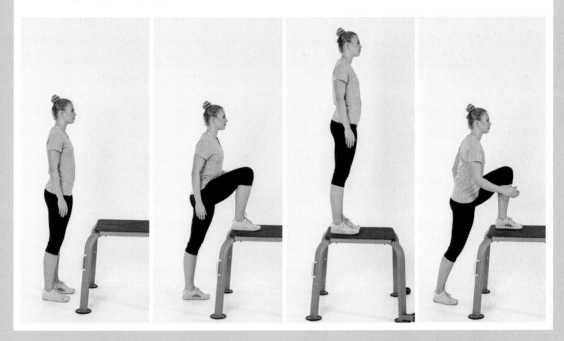

BOXING FORWARDS AND UPWARDS WHILE RUNNING ON THE SPOT

» Start with feet shoulder width apart, then run on the spot at a high tempo.

» As you do this, shadow-box in front of you and then straight up above your head, engaging your lats and shoulders as you do so. You are alternating between the two throughout the allotted time. Keep your abs tight to maintain balance. This exercise takes some coordination, but you will soon get the hang of it.

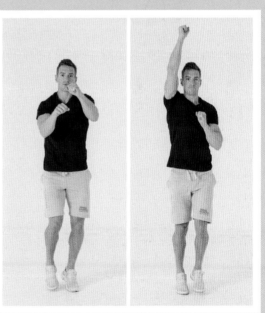

BOX JUMP

» Position a small box in front of you at knee height.

» Stand about 30cm away from it with your feet shoulder width apart.

» Squat down, then explode upwards and jump onto the box.

» When both feet are on the box, hop back down to the floor and descend into your squat. Repeat as required.

» Start slowly and build up your speed when doing jumps. You don't want to lose control.

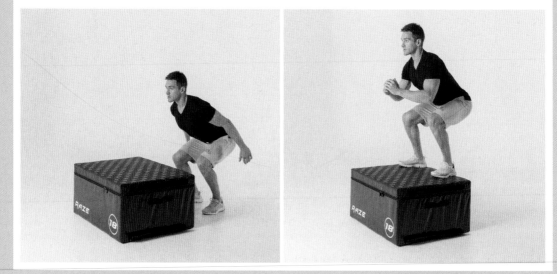

BOXING WHILE RUNNING ON THE SPOT

» Start with feet shoulder width apart, then run on the spot at a high tempo.

» As you do this, shadow-punch the air, engaging your lats and shoulders as you do so. Keep your abs tight to maintain balance. It's not a problem if you you rotate while running and punch in different directions.

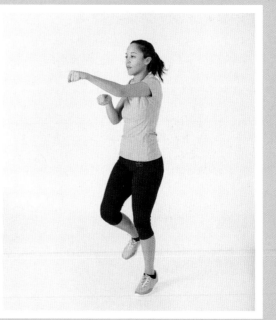

BOXING WITH SMALL DUMBBELLS

» Standing with your feet shoulder width apart, hold two small dumbbells and punch the air with them, using a variety of jabs, hooks and uppercuts.

» Stay on your toes and step from side to side, forward and back as you do this exercise.

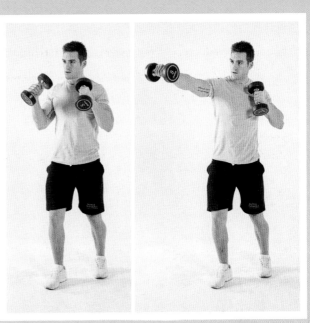

BREAK DANCER

» Start in a press-up position with your bodyweight distributed evenly between your hands and feet.

» Pivot onto your left arm and leg, letting your other leg and hand come up off the floor. The leg off the floor comes out in front of you. Return to the press-up position, but immediately pivot onto your right hand and right leg.

» Repeat as smoothly as possible.

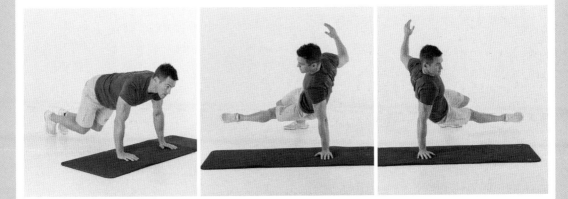

BROAD JUMP TO BACKWARD HOP

» Adopt an athletic position with your feet shoulder width apart, knees slightly bent and arms by your side.

» Bend at the knees and leap forward, landing on both feet. Focus on generating power, but do not go for a maximum effort jump as you need to keep your balance when you land.

» When you land, make sure you take the weight through your feet and bend your knees. You then hop backwards on both feet, using 3–4 small jumps to return to the starting position.

» Once back to the starting point, jump out again as far as you can.

» Don't rush these; take your time and build up speed. The more tired you get, the more you need to watch the backward hops.

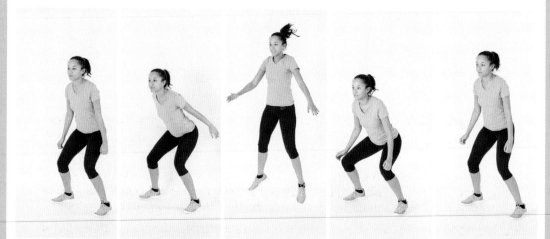

BULGARIAN SPLIT SQUAT

» Stand with a bench behind you, holding two dumbbells at your sides, or a barbell across your shoulders if you prefer.

» Lift your left foot back and place it on the bench behind you, with your weight resting on your toes or the ball of your foot. Keep your right foot firmly planted on the floor in front of you, adjusting it to a distance you find comfortable.

» Imagine you have a cable running through your head and straight through the middle of your body that is pulling you straight down, then drop the knee of the raised leg towards the floor, keeping your back straight. Squat down until your right hip is level with your right knee and you feel tension in your right glute. Ensure your knee does not track over your toes.

» Drive back upwards to the starting position.

» Unless stated otherwise, this exercise is always weighted. Where the bodyweight version is required, it is exactly the same but without the weights.

See pictures opposite »»»

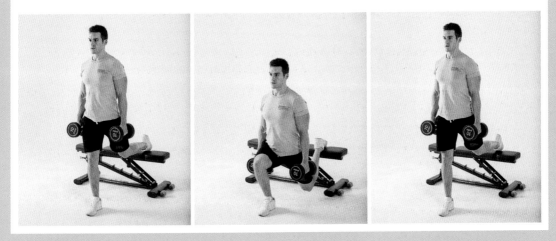

BURPEE

» Stand with your feet shoulder width apart, then drop onto your arms to adopt the top of a press-up position. Your legs will be shooting back behind you, so you take your weight more through your arms than your feet.

» Now explode back up to your feet, jumping upwards in one smooth movement. When doing this you are jumping your legs back underneath you and exploding off your hands. As you land, you do a small jump in the air and then try to land as quickly as possible.

» As your feet touch the floor, drop back down onto your front to adopt the start position of this exercise. This is a strict burpee.

» This is a great full-body conditioning exercise, so make sure you don't cheat when doing it. Every stage is equally important.

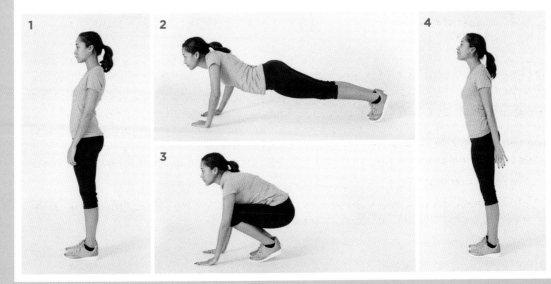

CABLE FACE-PULL

» Position a cable at face height and attach a rope grip. Hold the cable at arm's length in front of your face.

» Row the cable towards your face, bringing your elbows back, keeping them as high as possible and squeezing your shoulder blades together as you do so.

» Release the cable back to the starting position with control.

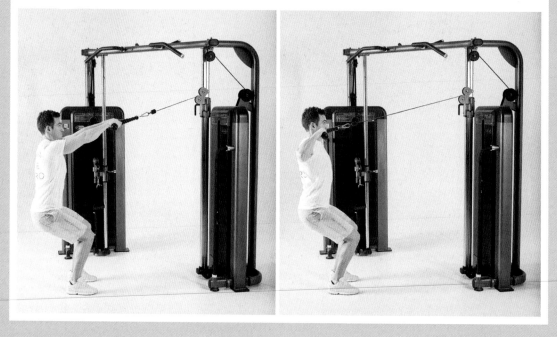

CABLE ROW

» If sitting on the floor, make sure your knees are slightly raised and soft. There are variously shaped handles you can use to do this exercise, and each will work slightly different muscles. If you are starting out, I suggest using a standard one.

» Reach forward and pull the cable into you, making sure you don't arch your back. Pull the cable into you as far as you can, take a pause and extend your arms back out as far as they go, using the full range at your disposal.

» If using a machine, select the appropriate weight, then sit on the seat in the position described above. Make sure you have a slight bend in your knees and that you don't arch backwards when pulling the cable towards you, or that you slump forward when lowering the weight.

» This exercise can be done either sitting on the floor or on a specialist cable row machine.

See pictures opposite » » »

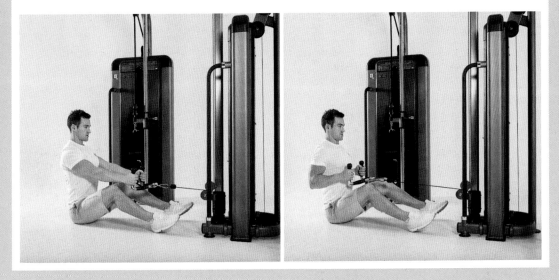

CALF RAISE

» Position you toes on a small block (at least 2.5cm) with your heel touching the floor.

» Push up onto your toes, then lower down. If this is too easy you can add some weights with some dumbbells (see page 118).

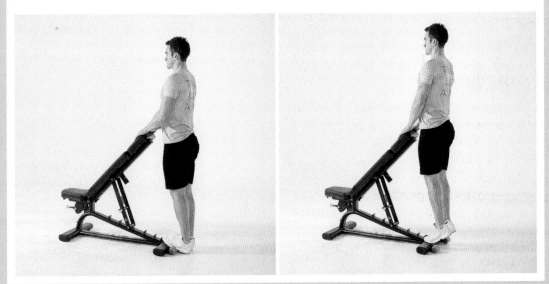

CARIOCA

» Adopt an athletic position with your feet shoulder width apart, your knees slightly bent and your arms bent at the elbow.

» The idea is to move sideways, crossing your legs over and behind one another as you do so. Choose your leading leg, i.e. if going to the right, you lead with your left leg. The left leg goes over your right foot, and then as you twist back, your left leg goes behind your right leg. Your right leg moves laterally. Use your arms to help you twist forward and back with the rotation of your leg.

» Perform 10 steps to the left, leading with the right leg, then do 10 steps to the right, leading with the left leg. Repeat as required.

» Make sure you rotate your upper body in conjunction with your legs. This is a whole body movement.

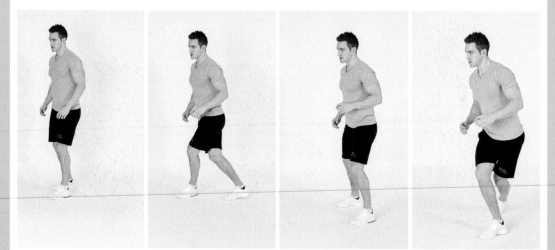

CHIN-UPS

» Grasp a chin-up bar with an underhand or neutral grip probably shoulder width apart. Allow your body to drop into a dead hang.

» Explode upwards towards the bar, bracing your abs and engaging your lats as you do so. If the instructions give you a slower tempo, make sure you pull up and lower as suggested.

» Make sure your chin clears the bar at the top, then lower yourself back down with control at the correct tempo. This phase is really important.

» Make sure your body doesn't swing or kip (i.e. arch or hollow to create momentum) when doing chin-ups of any kind. Swinging yourself up means you are not engaging the muscles properly.

Neutral grip

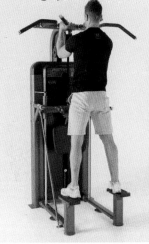
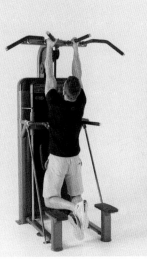
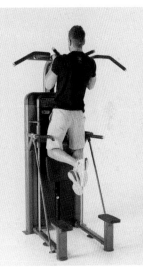

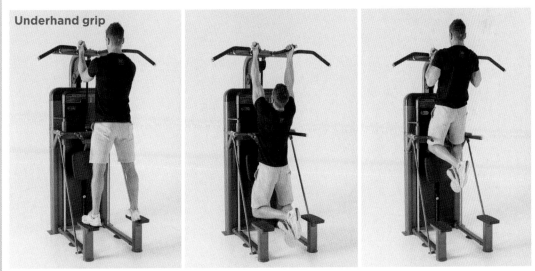

Underhand grip

COUNTERWEIGHT CHIN-UP

» Start by adjusting the machine to a weight that counterbalances your own.

» Grasp a chin-up bar with a neutral or underhand grip. Your knees will be resting on the counterweight pad of the machine.

» Explode (i.e. pull yourself) upwards towards the bar, bracing your abs and engaging your lats as you do so. The pad of the machine will come up with you as you go. If you find this too easy, you need to drop the counterweight so you are taking more of your own bodyweight.

» Make sure your chin clears the bar at the top without extending your neck, then lower yourself back down with control. This lowering phase is super-important.

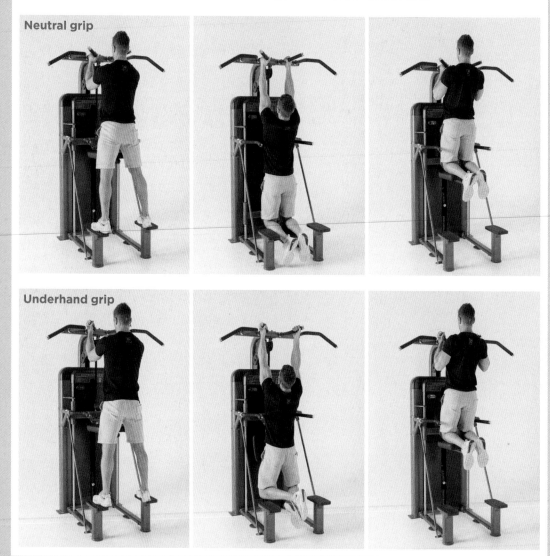

Neutral grip

Underhand grip

COUNTERWEIGHT DIP

» Set a counterbalance machine to the weight that counterbalances your bodyweight.

» Lower your body with control between the bars until your elbows are at right angles and your chest is level with the bars. Now explode back to the starting position, engaging your triceps and chest as you do so.

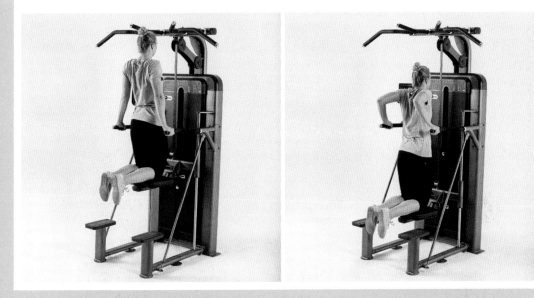

CROSS-TRAINER RUN

» Run at full capacity for the allotted time.

» Make sure you apply the correct amount of resistance to get the most from your workout.

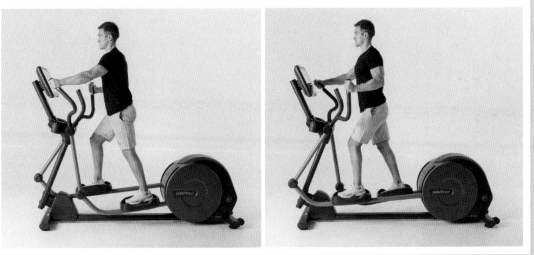

CURL TO PRESS

» Do not swing the dumbbells up. If you are doing this, the weight is too heavy. You need to control the weight or it will throw out the entire lift. To build muscle and size you must create tension in the muscles.

» Grasp two dumbbells in your hands and hold them by your sides.

» Keep your back straight at all times, bend your elbows to perform a bicep curl, bringing the dumbbells up to your shoulders. Do not hoist them up. As you curl the weight up, allow it to come forward a little to maintain tension in your bicep throughout the range of movement.

» At the top of the curl, transition into a shoulder press (see page 159) and lift the weights above your head. Ensure your arms are fully extended.

» Lower the weight with control back to the starting position.

» Stand or sit for this exercise, whichever feels more comfortable for you.

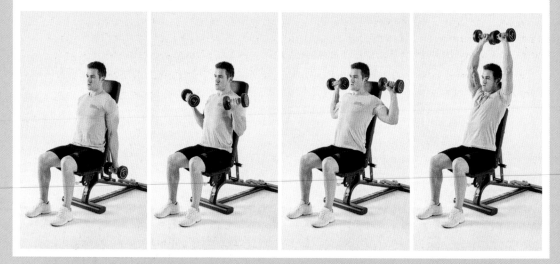

CURTSEY LUNGE

» Start from standing. Step your left leg behind you and to the right so that your thighs cross, bending both knees as if you are curtseying. Make sure your front knee is aligned with your front ankle.

» Return to standing, and repeat athe movement with your right leg behind you to complete one rep.

» Lunges are hard to master. Always focus on lunging out and down, not out and forward.

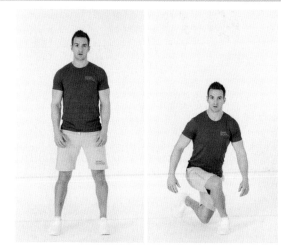

DEADLIFT

» When doing deadlifts, you need to warm up properly and make sure your technique is good every time. If you have any doubts, seek expert advice to teach you the right way.

» Stand facing a weighted barbell with your feet shoulder width apart. The barbell should be close to your shins.

» Sit back, place your weight in your heels and keep your back straight. Grasp the barbell with both hands, using an overhand grip (palms facing you), or an alternative grip as shown in the photos, whichever is more comfortable for you.

» Engage your abdominals, glutes and hamstrings and begin to lift the bar. As the bar travels up, keep it close to your shins at all times.

» Lift the bar until your legs and back are straight in a standing position, and push your hips forward slightly at the top of the movement. This will engage your glutes in a tense. Do not overthrust, however. Your spine should still be in line and you are not tucking under.

» Lower with control to the starting position, lightly touching the plates to the floor before repeating. During the lowering phase you will really feel your hamstrings working. Make sure you keep your back flat, shoulders back and chest out throughout the movement.

» When you reach the point of the hamstring extensions, it is important that you really engage your hamstrings and glutes, and do not allow your back to hinge.

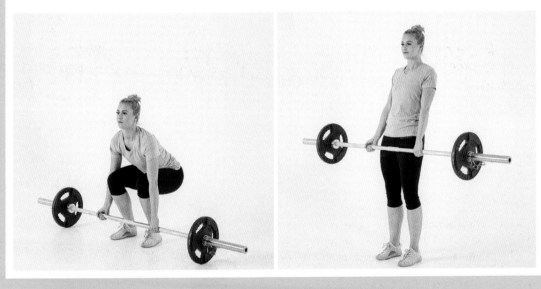

DECLINE DUMBBELL PRESS

» Position the base of a flat bench on a small block so that it sits at a slight decline or use a purpose built decline bench, as shown in the photos.

» Sit on the edge of the bench and grasp two dumbbells on your lap.

» Lie back and position the dumbbells just above your chest, with elbows bent. Ensure that your shoulders are pushed back and not internally rotated.

» Push the dumbbells up towards the ceiling until your arms are straight. The dumbbells should touch at the top of the movement.

» Focus on squeezing your chest muscles together as you push the dumbbells up.

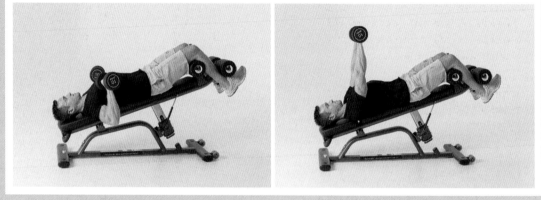

DECLINE PRESS-UP

» Start in a normal press-up position, with your feet elevated on a ledge or bench. Your hands should be shoulder width apart and level with your chest.

» Lower yourself as far as you can go without touching the floor, bracing your abs and keeping your back straight at all times. Drive back up to the start position.

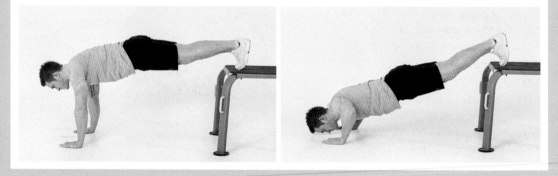

DIAGONAL ROTATIONAL CHOP

» Adopt an athletic position with your feet shoulder width apart and your knees slightly bent.

» Clasp your hands together and hold them out in front of you with fingers interlocked.

» Swing your arms explosively to the left and diagonally down, performing a chopping movement. Bring your arm back up, following the same diagonal to the right. Allow your feet to rotate to the side you are going and maintain tension in your abdominals.

» Do one set on your left, and one set on your right. Make sure you are fast and dynamic throughout.

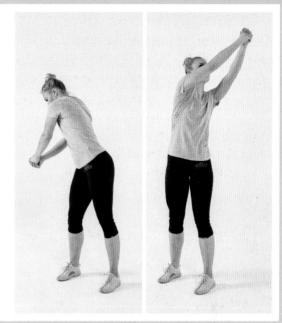

DIVE-BOMBER PRESS-UP

» Get on all fours on the floor with your feet hip width apart and hands shoulder width apart. Push your hips up as high as possible so that you resemble an inverted V. Keep your back flat with your arms and legs straight, but your knees unlocked.

» As you lower your hips, dive your upper body back down into a normal press, allowing your arms to bend as you push forward so that your chest nearly grazes the floor like a dive-bomber. You will end up coming forward over your hands, and your legs will be straight out, as in a normal press-up.

» Press back through your hands to full arm extension, drive your hips back upwards, and straighten your legs, reforming the V. Repeat as required.

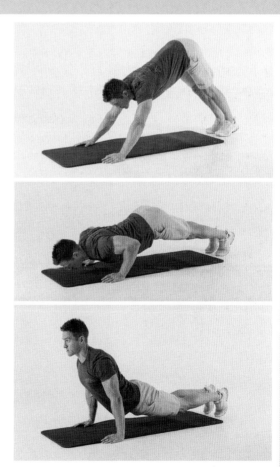

DONKEY CALF-RAISE

» Stand with your toes on small block (at least 2.5cm thick) with your heels touching the floor.

» Bend forward at the hips and hold onto something sturdy.

» Raise yourself up on tiptoes, then slowly lower down again.

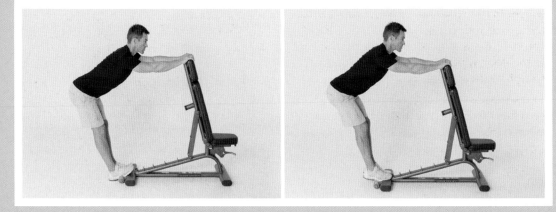

DOWN AND UP

» This is different from a burpee, as you are going completely to the floor and there is no jump on the way back up.

» Stand tall, then drop your chest and body to the floor as quickly as you can and return to standing as fast and dynamically as possible. The idea is to let your entire body touch the floor, then to bounce back to your feet.

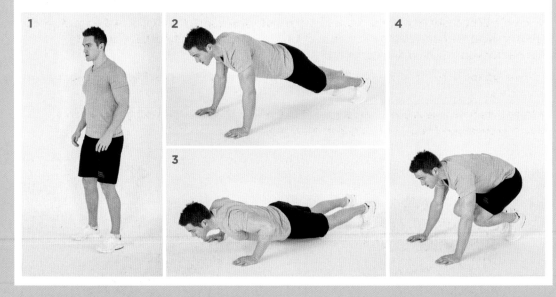

DROP SQUAT

» Stand with your feet, slightly wider than, shoulder width apart in a relaxed position, then start shuffling your feet in a slow run.

» Every 2 seconds, drop into a squat as follows: making sure you have all your weight in your heels, quickly drop to the bottom of your squat position by jumping your feet out and dropping your bottom to the floor, while maintaining a good straight back and head up.

» Power back up to standing, using your hamstrings, glutes and hips. Repeat as required.

» In this exercise it's important to keep moving the whole time.

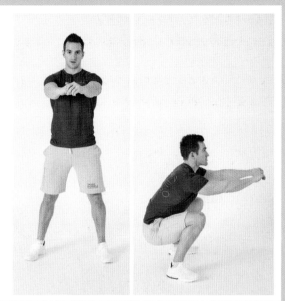

DUMBBELL BENCH PRESS

» Sit on the edge of a bench and grasp two dumbbells on your lap.

» Lie back and position the dumbbells just above your chest, with elbows bent. Ensure that your shoulders are pushed back and not internally rotated.

» Push the dumbbells up, towards the ceiling until your arms are straight, taking the recommended 4 seconds to do so. The dumbbells should touch at the top of the movement.

» Focus on squeezing your chest muscles together as you push the dumbbells to the ceiling.

» Lower the dumbbells with control over a period of 4 seconds (the tempo will vary from week to week). Return to the starting position, then push the weights back upwards. Repeat for your allotted number of reps.

» Never go too low on the way down doing dumbbell press. They should stop just above your chest.

» Make sure you always use a full range of motion with this exercise, taking the weights down to chest level and extending all the way up.

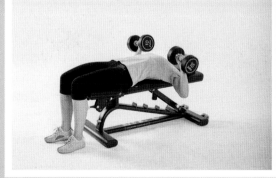
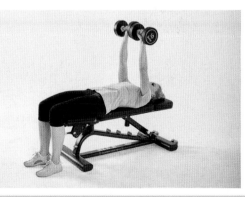

DUMBBELL BENT-OVER ROW

» Adopt an athletic position with your knees slightly bent. Pick two dumbbells up from the floor with an overhand grip.

» Bend at the knees until you are just above horizontal, keeping your back flat and your weight in your heels.

» Keeping your back straight, row the weight towards your chest just below your sternum. Focus on squeezing your shoulder blades together as you do this to engage your back muscles.

» Lower the dumbbells with control to the starting position.

» Make sure you keep your head neutral when doing a bent-over row. Too many people arch their neck. Find a spot on the floor just in front of you and focus on it while you lift.

DUMBBELL CALF-RAISE

» Holding two dumbbells in your hands, position your toes on a small block or plate (at least 2.5cm thick), with your heels touching the floor.

» Push up and then lower slowly at the allocated tempo

DUMBBELL FLY

» Lie back on a bench and hold the dumbbells in a neutral grip just above your chest, with elbows bent. Your palms are facing each other when holding the dumbbells up and out in front of you.

» Slowly lower the dumbbells out to the side, feeling the tension in your chest.

» When they are just above parallel, slowly bring them up and touch together at the top. Repeat as required.

» Your arms should never straighten in this exercise. Do not let them come out too low to your sides. The dumbbells should never go lower than your body. You need to maintain tension in your chest as you do this exercise.

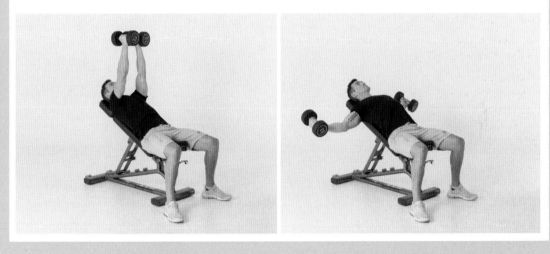

DUMBBELL REVERSE CURL

» While standing, hold the dumbbells at your side with your palms facing you.

» Curl the weight upwards, but do not turn your wrist. At the top of the movement your palms should be facing away. You should feel the tension in your forearms.

» Lower the weight with control and repeat.

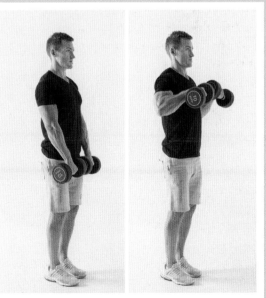

DUMBBELL ROMANIAN DEADLIFT

» Pick the dumbbells off the floor using the deadlift technique on page 115. Hold the dumbbells at hip level with a pronated (palms facing down) grip or an alternative grip. Your shoulders should be back, your back arched, and your knees slightly bent.

» Lower the dumbbells by moving your butt back as far as you can. Keep the bar close to your body, your head looking forward and your shoulders back. Done correctly, you should reach the maximum range of your hamstring flexibility just below the knee. Any further movement will be compensation and should be avoided for this movement. You will have a slight bend in your knees when you are lowering. Make sure to keep your back flat and your head neautral.

» At the bottom of your range of motion, return to the starting position by driving the hips forward to stand up tall. You should feel an increase in tension in your glutes.

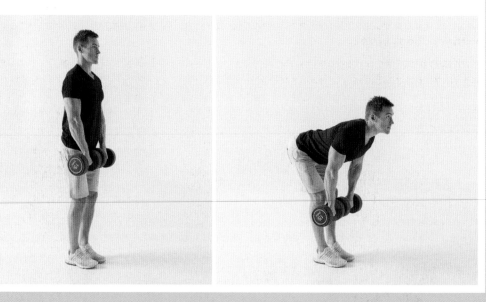

DUMBBELL STEP-UP

» Stand with your feet shoulder width apart, facing a bench or box set to a height just above your knees.

» Hold two dumbbells in your hands with an overhand grip.

» Using your left leg, step onto the bench, then follow with your right leg so that both feet are planted on the bench. You can drive your free knee through so that you finish at the top of the movement with one leg on the box and one knee at 90 degrees or stand with both feet on the box.

» Lower the left leg to the floor, then follow with your right leg so that both feet are now back on the ground. Make sure you engage your glutes on the way down.

» Repeat the process, this time leading with your right leg.

» To make this exercise harder you can increase the height of the bench or box or add more weight. If you don't feel confident enough to do this weighted, just keep working with your bodyweight.

» Always focus on engaging your glutes, or bottom muscles, as you power up and lower down. You should always have tension in this area.

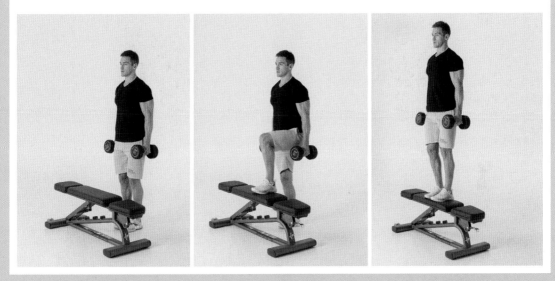

DUMBBELL SQUAT

» Hold the dumbbells out to your sides, with your feet shoulder width apart.

» Lower your bottom to the floor in a controlled manner while maintaining a flat back. You want to have your weight through your heels the entire time, keeping your back straight and your head level.

» When you get as low as your body will let you, use your hamstrings and glutes to drive you back up.

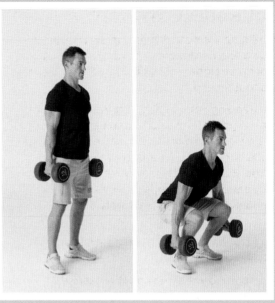

DUMBBELL THRUSTER

» Adopt an athletic position with your feet shoulder width apart.

» Using a neutral grip, hold two dumbbells that you can comfortably press overhead at your shoulders.

» Squat down, keeping your back straight and your weight in your heels.

» Drive up and, as you do so, press the weights overhead.

» Return the weights to the starting position and repeat.

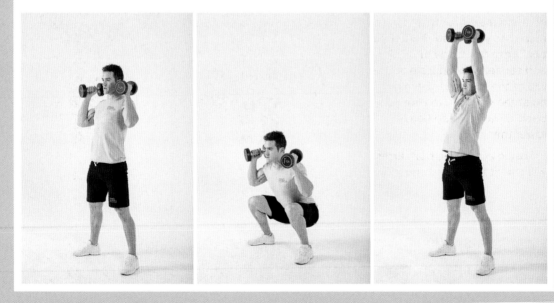

DUMBBELL UPRIGHT ROW

» Grasp your dumbbell with an overhand grip and hold them in front of your thighs, arms straight. Your grip should be roughly shoulder width apart.

» Keeping your back straight at all times, raise your elbows up and to the side to lift the weights to the top of your chest. Keep the bar close to your body as you raise it. You should feel this movement in your upper back and traps. If necessary, you can put one foot in front of the other to balance yourself.

» Lower the weights with control to the starting position.

» Do not do half-reps on this exercise. Control the barbell or kettlebell all the way from bottom to top, making sure your elbows travel up first.

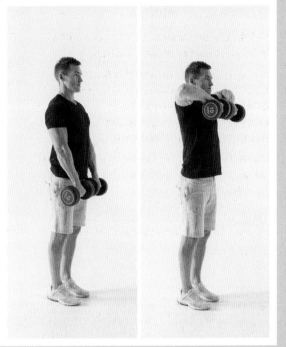

EZ BAR CURL

» While standing, grasp an EZ bar in your hands. Keep your back straight and your feet planted firmly on the ground.

» Curl the bar towards your chest, creating maximal tension in your biceps as you do so. Ensure you perform a full range of motion and squeeze the muscle at the top of the movement. Do not hoist the weights up with your back. If they are too heavy, lower the weight.

» If using an EZ bar, both arms will curl at the same time.

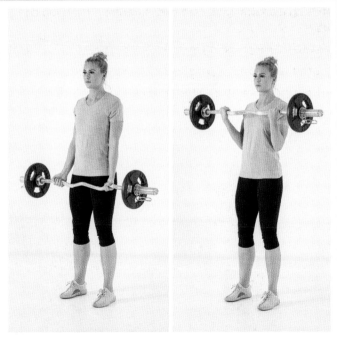

EZ BAR REVERSE CURL

» While standing, hold an EZ bar straight bar with an overhand grip.

» Curl the weight upwards, but do not turn your wrist. At the top of the movement your palms should be facing away. You should feel the tension in your forearms.

» Lower the weight with control and repeat.

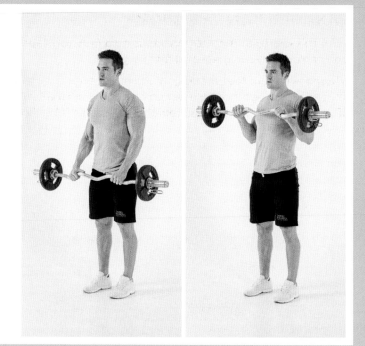

EZ BAR SKULL-CRUSHER

» Standing or lying flat on a bench, hold an EZ bar above your head with a neutral grip, arms straight. Alternatively, grasp a dumbbell between two hands above your head in a vice grip.

» Keeping your back straight and your abs tight, slowly lower the bar or dumbbell until it's over your head, just above your forehead (hence the name skull-crusher).

» Push upwards back to the starting position as you exhale. When your arms are again fully extended above your head you have completed one rep.

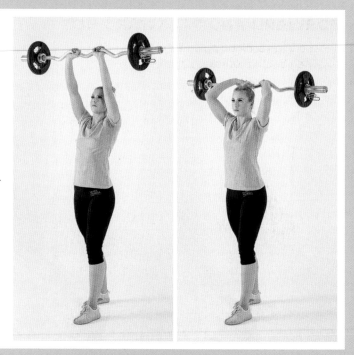

FAST FEET ON THE SPOT

» For this exercise, imagine you are using a footwork ladder and can't raise your knees and feet very high.

» Stand with your feet shoulder width apart, then run on the spot at the highest possible tempo but using minimal knee lift. You want the smallest possible movements off the floor.

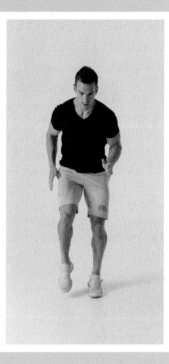

FORWARD AND BACKWARD HOP ON THE SPOT

» Stand in an athletic position, with your feet shoulder width apart. Jump both feet forward and then back as quickly as you can.

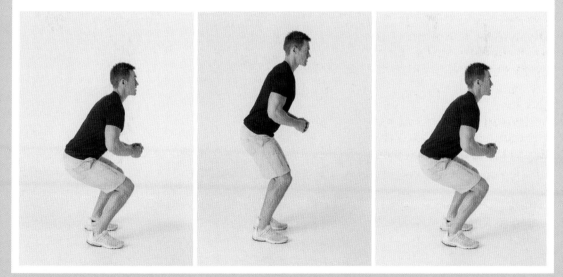

FORWARD LUNGE

» Stand tall with your feet hip width apart and engage your core.

» Take a big step forward with your left leg, then start to shift your weight forward so the heel hits the floor first.

» Lower your body until your left thigh is parallel to the floor and your left shin is vertical (it's okay if the knee shifts forward a little, as long as it doesn't go past the left toe). If your mobility allows, lightly tap the right knee to ground while keeping your weight in the left heel. Imagine you have a weight pulling you down from your middle, so you lunge out and down, not out and forward.

» Press into the left heel to drive back up to starting position. You are not moving forward

» Repeat the movement on the other side.

FRONT PLANKS

» Adopt a press-up position with your hands shoulder width apart and your weight supported on your forearms, bent at the elbow. (You can do the plank in a straight-arm form as well.)

» Brace your abs to balance, keeping your back straight at all times and your glutes high. Your body should be perfectly straight as you hold this position.

» Hold for 20–30 seconds, then come out of the plank onto your knees and rest as specified before repeating.

» Do not let your middle sag when doing the plank. Engage your abs and buttocks throughout.

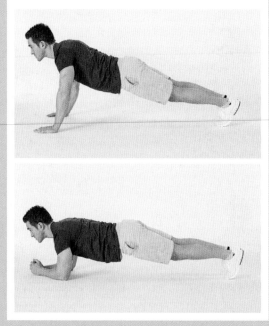

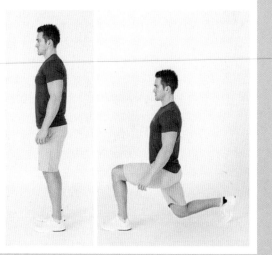

FRONT PLANK WITH HAND TAP

» Adopt a secure front plank position, then lift your right hand off the floor to touch your left hand, then return it to the starting position, then touch your left hand to your right hand in the same way. Now repeat, with your left hand touching your right hand.

» Continue to tap each hand alternately, maintaining perfect posture and abdominal tension.

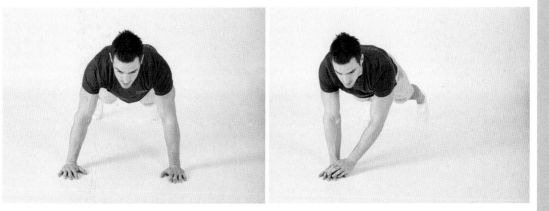

FULL BODY CRUNCH

» Although abdominal exercises have to be done dynamically, it is a common mistake to do them too fast. Take this exercise at a steady pace.

» Remember too that although this exercise is done lying down, your arms and feet should never rest on the floor during the working set or you will lose tension in your body.

» Lie on the floor, legs out straight, with your hands stretched out over your head.

» Bring your knees and chest together, lifting them simultaneously and maintaining abdominal tension. Your arms go out straight to the side of your legs. The only thing left resting on the floor should be your bottom.

» Lower with control until your neck and feet are a few centimetres off the floor, and your arms and legs are both stretched out once again. Repeat as required.

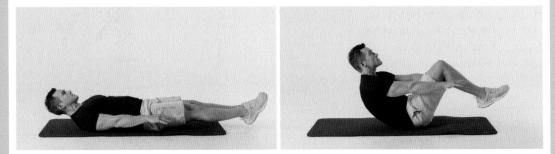

GLUTE BRIDGE

» Really engage your glutes throughout this movement. Make sure you go all the way down and all the way up: you do not want just short thrusts.

» Lie on your back with your feet on the floor and your knees bent, pointing towards the ceiling. However, you are never resting in the bottom position. Maintain tension in your glutes.

» Keeping your weight in your heels, drive your hips upwards, contracting your glutes as you do so. Drive until your back is straight and your hips are level with your knees.

» Lower your trunk back to the floor with control. Touch the floor gently with your glutes, then contract them again to thrust back upwards.

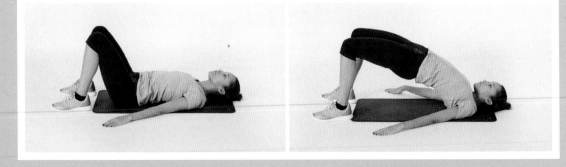

GOBLET SQUAT

» Stand with your feet, slightly wider than, shoulder width apart, holding a dumbbell or kettlebell vertically at your chest, like a goblet. Your hands will be either under the end of a dumbbell or around the bell part of a kettlebell.

» Lower down into a squat position, keeping your abs tight and your back straight. Remember to go only as low as you can while maintaining perfect form. This means ensuring that your knees track out rather than buckling in, and that your back does not arch.

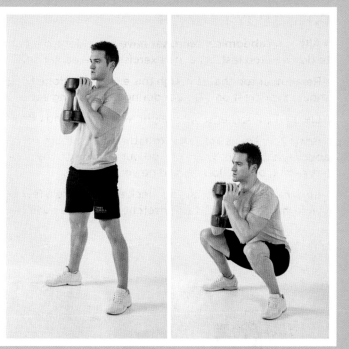

HALO SLAM

» Stand with your feet shoulder width apart and adopt an athletic position, knees slightly bent.

» Clasp your hands together in a tight grip, interlocking your fingers, and put them out in front of you, arms straight.

» Lift your arms above your head and to your right, keeping your abs and glutes engaged. As you do this, your knees should straighten. Circle your arms around your head in a halo shape, then hold them at the top of your head.

» When your arms are fully extended, brace your core, bend at the knees and slam your arms down to the starting position. You should maintain full abdominal tension throughout this movement. You then return to the start position and circle the other way, mimicking a halo.

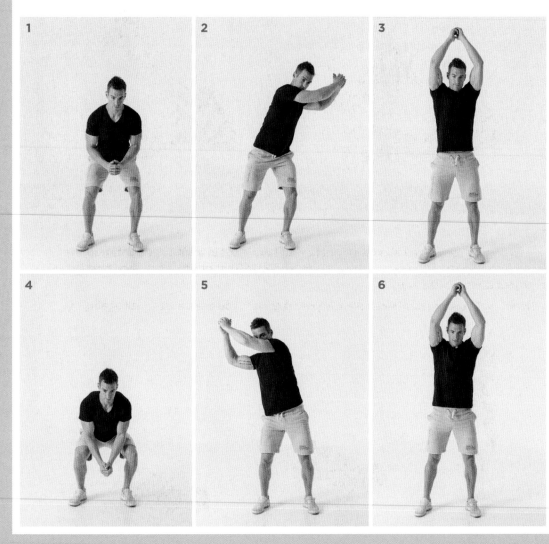

HAMSTRING EXTENSION

There are many types of hamstring extension machine. Whichever you have access to, it's really important to engage your hamstrings and glutes the whole time. You do not want to overload your lower back or overhinge at the hips.

» Stand with your feet locked in place and hinge from your waist, making sure to keep your back flat and your head neutral.

» It's also important to raise and lower with control. Do not use momentum to swing you back into standing.

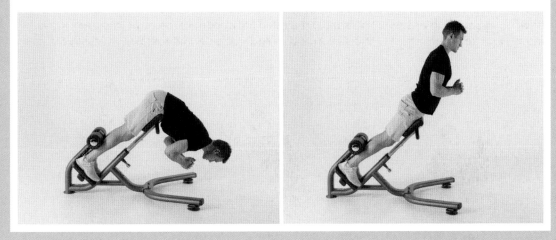

HAMSTRING WALKOUTS

» Standing tall, bend over slowly and walk your hands out in front of you until you are in a press-up position, your arms slightly extended in front of you, your back straight and your abdominals tight.

» Slowly walk your hands back towards your feet until you are standing tall again.

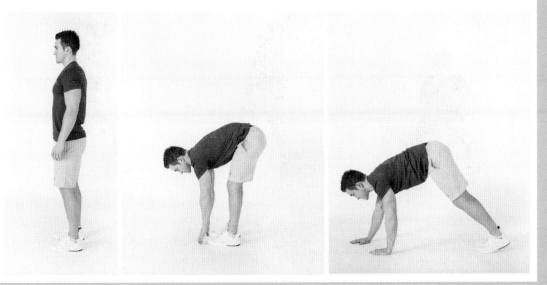

IN-AND-OUT SQUAT

» Start with your feet shoulder width apart, then lower down into a squat, taking the weight through your heels.

» In this position, jump your feet in and out while maintaining the squat. Do this as dynamically as possible.

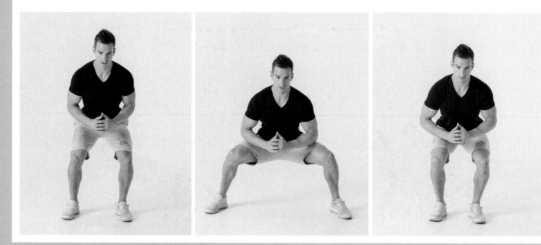

INCLINE DUMBBELL FLY

» Position a weight bench to a 45° incline. Lie on the bench on your back with two light dumbbells in your hands, holding them out to the side in an arc. Your elbows should be bent and your palms facing inwards. You should feel a light stretch in your chest.

» Squeeze your chest muscles to bring the weights up in a half-moon shape so that they touch directly above your head. Your elbows should remain slightly bent to avoid stress on the biceps.

» Slowly lower the weights back to the starting position with control.

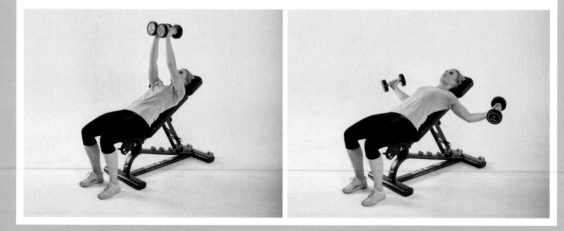

INCLINE DUMBBELL PRESS

» Position a weight bench to a 30-degree incline. Sit on the edge of the bench and grasp two dumbbells on your lap. Lie back and position the dumbbells just above your chest, with elbows bent. Ensure that your shoulders are pushed back and not internally rotated.

» Push the dumbbells up towards the ceiling until your arms are straight. The dumbbells should touch at the top of the movement.

» Focus on squeezing your chest muscles together as you push the dumbbells to the ceiling.

» Lower the dumbbells with control. Return to the starting position, then push back upwards.

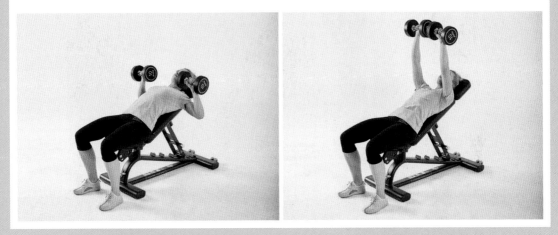

INCLINE DUMBBELL REVERSE ROW

» Position a weight bench to a 45-degree incline. Lie face down on the bench, hang your arms by your sides and hold two dumbbells in your hands.

» Row these dumbbells up one at a time (as shown in the photos) or together until level with your chest, ensuring you feel the tension in your lats and upper back. Lower with control.

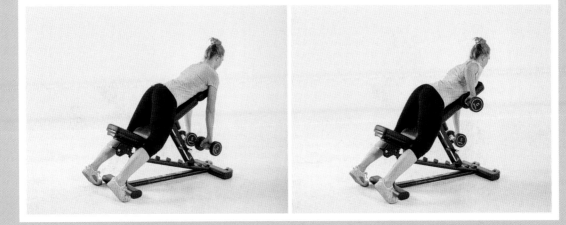

INCLINE PRESS-UP

» Place a small bench or ledge at least 30cm off the floor. Adopt a normal press-up position, with your hands shoulder width apart on the bench or ledge and your feet on the floor. Your bodyweight should be distributed equally between your hands and feet.

» Lower yourself down as far as you can go without letting your chest touch the box or ledge. Make sure you are bracing your abs and keeping your back straight at all times. Drive back up to the start position.

» To engage your chest muscles, imagine that you are pushing your hands together while you are doing the press-up.

» If you don't get the set-up right for incline press-ups, they can become easy. Make sure you are constantly testing yourself.

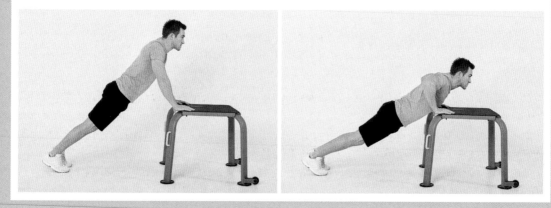

INCLINE REVERSE LATERAL RAISE

» Position an adjustable bench to a 45° incline when measured from the floor.

» Lie face down on the bench and hang your arms downwards, elbows slightly bent, holding a dumbbell in each hand.

» As you exhale, raise your arms out to the side until your elbows are at shoulder height and your arms are roughly parallel to the floor. Keep the contraction at the top for a second.

» Slowly lower the dumbbells to the starting position as you inhale.

» Repeat as required.

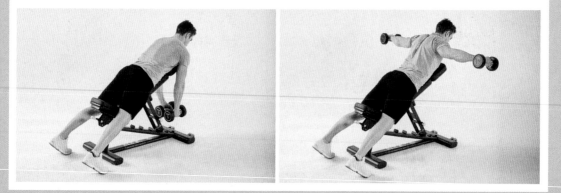

JUMPING MOUNTAIN CLIMBER

» Start in a traditional press-up position, but with your feet slightly further apart than normal.

» Taking your weight through your hands, jump both feet inwards so that your knees come up under your chest.

» Jump your feet back. Repeat dynamically.

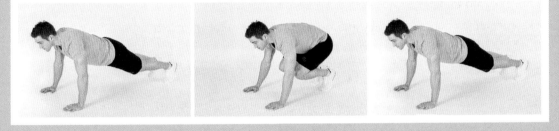

KETTLEBELL STANDING CLEAN TO PRESS

» Stand in an athletic position, holding a kettlebell in your right hand by your side in an overhand grip.

» 'Clean' the kettlebell by lifting it up to your shoulders, using your legs and hips to drive it up. Keep your palm facing outwards and do not 'curl' the kettlebell.

» As the the kettlebell travels up, it will rotate, so the bell part will be sitting against the front of your arm.

» Press the kettlebell overhead until your arm is fully extended. Reverse this motion to return to the starting position with control. The kettlebell will swing around to the position in which it started. Repeat with the left hand.

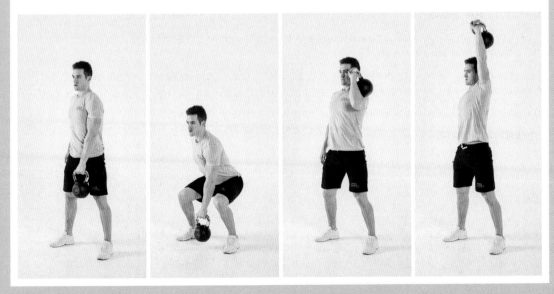

KETTLEBELL SWING

» Stand in an athletic position, arms by your sides, holding a kettlebell between your legs.

» Drop down into a half-squat position, then use your hips to drive the kettlebell forward. Swing it up so that it is level with your face, your legs and hips are driving the weight up.

» Drop back down, bending at the knees as the kettlebell comes down, and let it swing between your legs. Maintain a continuous swinging motion, engaging your hips and using your glutes to drive the bell forward and maintain balance. You should feel this exercise in your core, glutes, hamstrings and shoulders.

» Do not use your arms or upper body to swing the kettlebell up.

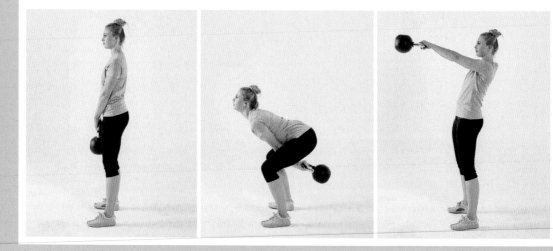

KETTLEBELL UPRIGHT ROW

» Grasp your kettlebell with an overhand grip and hold it in front of your thighs, arms straight.

» Keeping your back straight at all times, raise your elbows up and to the side to lift the kettlebell to the top of your chest. Keep the kettlebell close to your body as you raise it. You should feel this movement in your upper back and traps. If necessary, you can put one foot in front of the other to balance yourself.

» Lower the kettlebell with control to the starting position.

» Do not do half-reps on this exercise. Control the kettlebell all the way from bottom to top, making sure your elbows travel up first.

See pictures opposite » » »

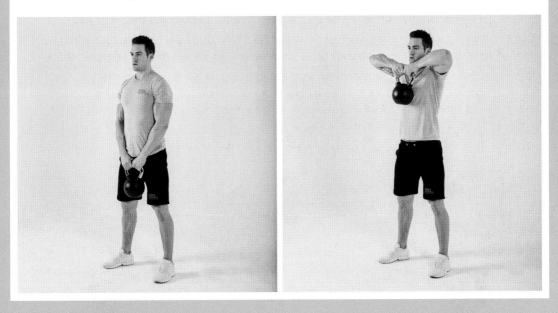

KNEELING PRESS-UP

» Kneel on the floor with your back flat and your toes shoulder width apart and level with your chest. The further you have your knees back, the harder the press-up will be. For even greater intensity, you can cross your feet.

» Lower yourself down as far as possible without touching the floor. Drive back up to the starting position and repeat.

» Imagine pushing your hands together while doing the press-up to engage your chest muscle.

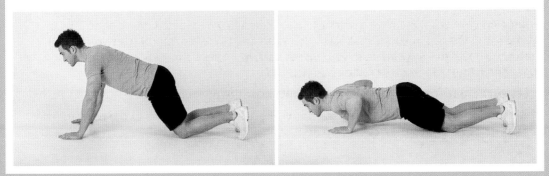

KNEELING NARROW HAND PLACEMENT PRESS-UP

» Perform a press-up as above with hands narrower than shoulder width.

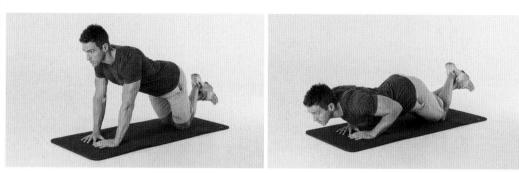

KNEELING WIDE HAND HAND PLACEMENT PRESS-UP

» Perform a press-up as above with hands wider than shoulder width.

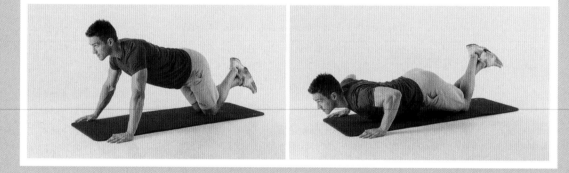

LATERAL LUNGE

» Start from standing. Step out to the right and shift your body weight over your right leg, squatting to a 90-degree angle at the right knee. Try to sit down on your butt, keeping your back as upright as possible.

» Push off and bring your right leg back to the centre to complete one rep.

» Repeat the movement on the left side.

See pictures opposite » » »

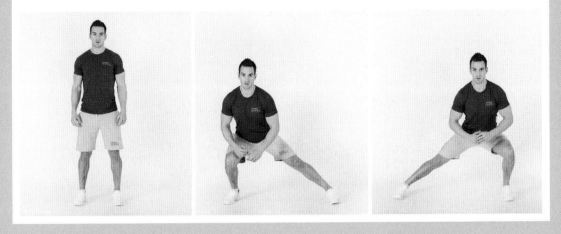

LATERAL PULL-DOWN

» This targets the same muscles as chin-ups.

» Sit at a lat pull-down machine with your knees under the cushion.

» With hands shoulder width apart, grasp the weighted bar above you in an underhand grip, then pull it down to your chest in a smooth movement.

» Equally smoothly, let the bar travel back upwards to the start position.

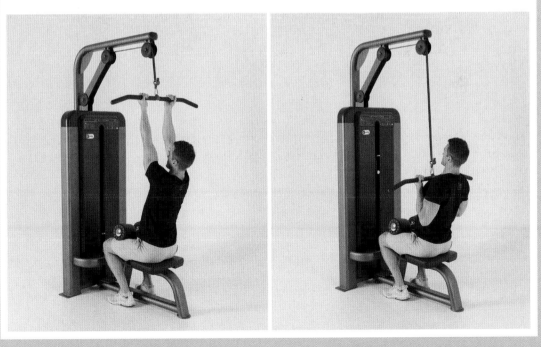

LEG EXTENSION

» Position yourself on a leg extension machine. Align the pad with the bottom of your shins, just above your feet.

» Raise your legs against the pad for the full range of motion until they are straight. Maintain crisp form throughout the movement. Make sure the eccentric and concentric phases are done at the appropriate tempo. (The tempo will change for certain weeks.)

» This exercise is about control. Make sure you always take a 1-second pause at the top of the movement. Do not go too fast.

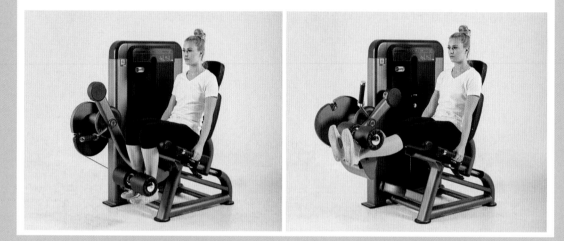

LEG PRESS

» Seated on a leg press machine, position your feet roughly shoulder width apart. Press down hard on the platform, engaging your quads, hamstrings and calves as you do so. Release the latch so that you take full control of the weight.

» Push out until your legs are straight. Ensure you do not lock your knees at the top of the movement. Lower the weight with control, going as low as possible without putting too much pressure on your lower back and without compromising your form. Repeat as required.

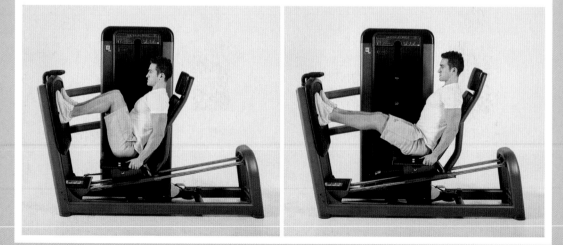

LOW ROTATIONAL CHOP

» This movement is the same as a rotational chop, but here you are in a squat position.

» Adopt an athletic position, with your feet shoulder width apart and your knees slightly bent. Clasp your hands together with your fingers interlocked and hold them directly out in front of you.

» Drop down into a small squat and swing your arms explosively to the right-hand side, keeping a low centre of gravity and performing a chopping movement.

» Rotate quickly back to the left.

» Allow your feet to dynamically rotate as you chop from side to side.

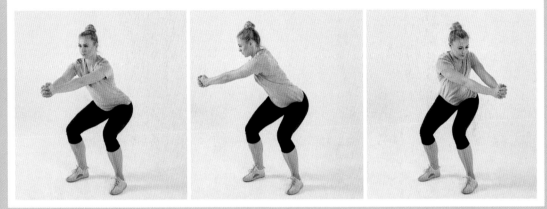

LUNGE CHANGE-UP

» Stand in an athletic position with your feet shoulder width apart. Perform a reverse lunge by stepping backwards with your right foot and bending at the knee.

» At the bottom of your lunge, explode upwards, bringing your right leg back up. Drive it through the starting position and bring your knee up to your chest.

» Return your left leg to the starting position and repeat on the left-hand side.

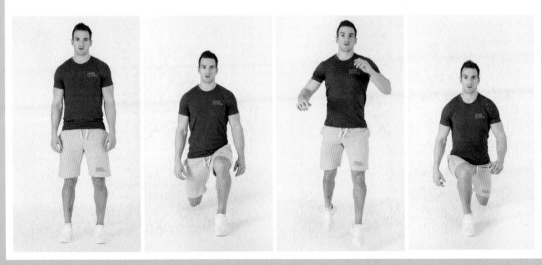

MACHINE-ASSISTED CALF-RAISE

» Position your lower hips and back under the padded lever, your arms on the side handles and the balls of your feet on the calf block, with the heels extending off.

» Raise your heels as you push up onto your toes, extending your ankles as far as possible. Ensure the knee is kept stationary at all times.

» Hold the contracted position for a second before lowering your heels with control to the starting position.

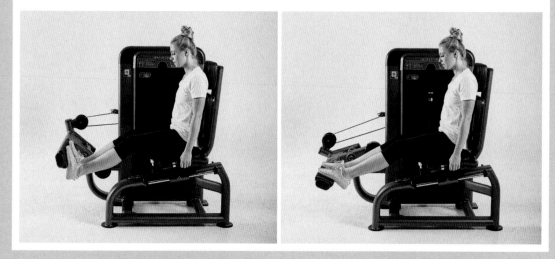

MACHINE ASSISTED HAMSTRING CURL

» There are a number of different machines for performing hamstring curls, which can be done either while lying prone, seated, or while standing. As I don't know what machine you will be using, the description below is for lying hamstring curls. Try to use an angled leg curl machine as opposed to a flat one, since the angled position is more favourable for engaging the hamstrings. Make sure you find the right weight on your chosen machine and go through the full controlled range of movement.

» Adjust the machine lever to fit your height and lie face down on the leg curl machine with the pad of the lever on the back of your legs (just a few centimetres under the calves).

» Keeping the torso flat on the bench, ensure your legs are fully stretched and your toes straight, and grab the side handles of the machine.

» As you exhale, curl your legs up as far as possible without lifting the upper legs from the pad. Once you hit the fully contracted position, hold it for a second.

» As you inhale, bring the legs back to the start position. Repeat as required.

» The photos opposite show a seated hamstring curl.

See pictures opposite » » »

»»» Machine assisted hamstring curl

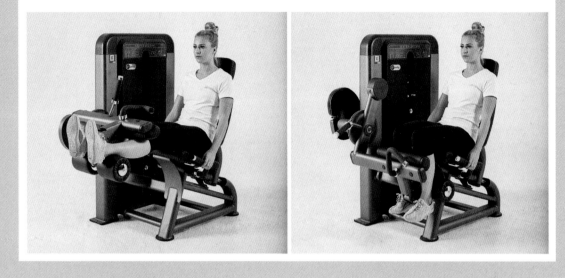

MACHINE PRESS

» Sit down on the chest press machine and select the weight.

» Make sure the handles are in line with your chest, then hold them with a palms-down grip and lift your elbows so that your upper arms are parallel to the floor.

» As you exhale and flex your pecs, push the handles forward and extend your arms straight in front of you. Hold the contraction for a second.

» Now bring the handles back towards you as you breathe in.

» Repeat as required.

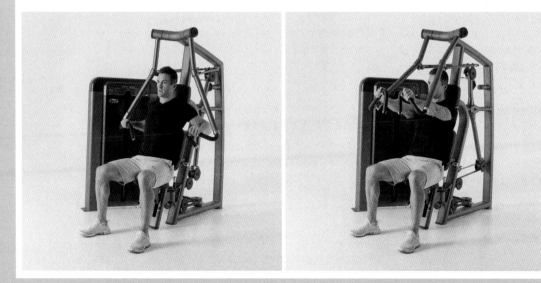

MACHINE ROWS

» Adjust the seat so that the handles are at chest level.

» Slowly pull the handles towards your chest, engaging yuor shoulder blades as you flex the elbow.

» Slowly return the handles to the starting position.

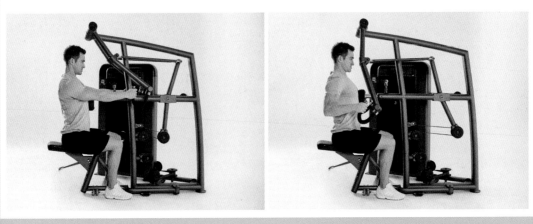

MEDICINE BALL HALO SLAM

» Stand with your feet shoulder width apart and adopt an athletic position, knees slightly bent holding a medicine ball.

» Clasp a medicine ball and hold it out in front of you, arms straight.

» Lift the ball above your head and to your right, keeping your abs and glutes engaged. As you do this, your knees should straighten. Circle the ball around your head in a halo shape, then hold the ball above your head.

» When your arms are fully extended, brace your core, bend at the knees and slam the ball into the ground as hard as possible. You should maintain full abdominal tension throughout this movement. Pick the ball up again, or catch it if it bounces and circle the other way, mimicking a halo.

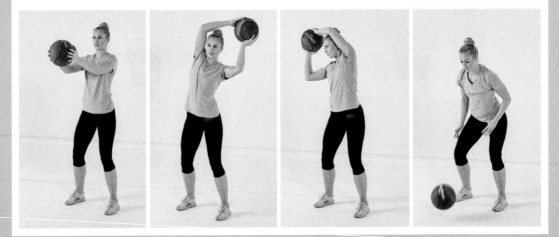

MEDICINE BALL SLAM

» Stand in an athletic position holding a medicine ball. Lift the ball above your head, arms fully extended, then slam the ball down onto the floor as hard as you can.

» Squat down to pick the ball up, keeping your back straight and abs tight. Often the ball bounces so you can catch it on the way back up. Return to starting position and repeat for your total work time.

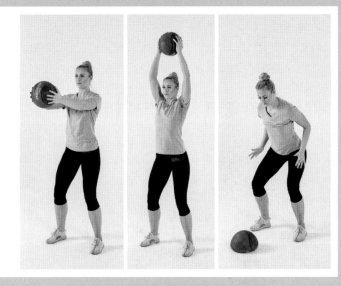

MILITARY PRESS

» Stand in an athletic position with your feet shoulder width apart, one foot slightly in front of the other and your knees slightly bent. Hold a barbell at chest level, your palms facing away from you and all four fingers and thumb on the same side of the bar.

» Press the bar upwards above your head until your arms are fully extended. Keep your abs and glutes tight as you press and do not arch your back. Your feet should remain firmly on the floor. If they are not, you are lifting too heavy.

» Lower the bar back to your chest with control, then repeat as required.

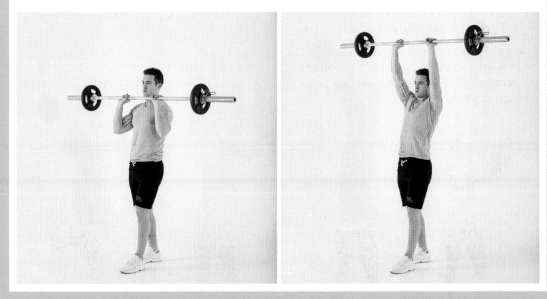

MOUNTAIN CLIMBER

» Start slowly and build up your speed when doing mountain climbers. You don't want to lose control. Do this exercise at a steady pace, slower than running, and maintain maximum abdominal tension throughout.

» Adopt a press-up position, with your weight evenly distributed between your hands and feet. Your feet should be slightly further apart than normal.

» Taking your weight through your hands, move your right foot forward, bringing your knee into your chest. Drive the raised knee back, while bringing up the other knee.

» Your legs should pump forwards and back in a continuous fluid motion, the aim being to get the full range with each movement.

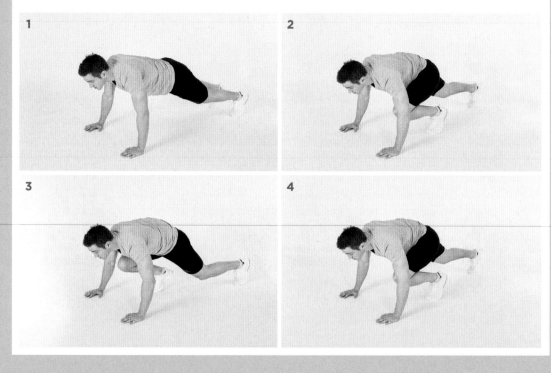

MOUNTAIN CLIMBER TO BURPEE

» Do the mountain climber as described opposite, but every 5 seconds leap to your feet and spring off the floor to perform a burpee. Drop back down into the starting position and continue your mountain climbers.

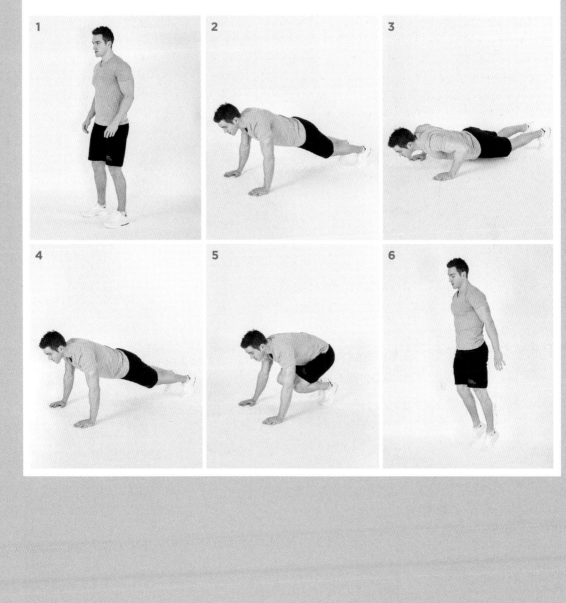

NARROW HAND PLACEMENT PRESS-UPS

» Hold yourself in a front plank position, with your hands narrower than shoulder width apart and level with your chest.

» Lower yourself down as far as possible without touching the floor. Drive back up to the starting position and repeat.

» Imagine pushing your hands together while doing the press-up to engage your chest muscles.

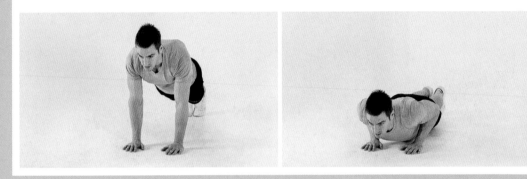

NARROW WALL PRESS-UPS

» Keeping your arms straight, place your hands next to each other against a wall.

» Slowly lower your face to the wall, getting as close as you can without touching it. The further back you get your feet, the harder it is.

» Push out again, then repeat as required.

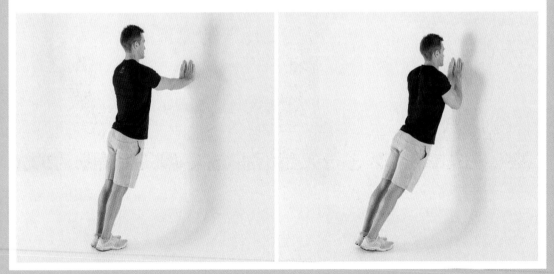

PRESS-UPS

» Press-ups should always be done in a controlled manner. You want to go through the full range of motion at your disposal – we don't want any half-reps.

» Get yourself into a normal press-up position, hands shoulder width apart and level with your chest. Your weight should be evenly spread between your hands and feet.

» Lower yourself down as far as possible without actually touching the floor. Drive back up to the start position and repeat.

» Imagine pushing your hands together while doing the press-up to engage your chest muscles.

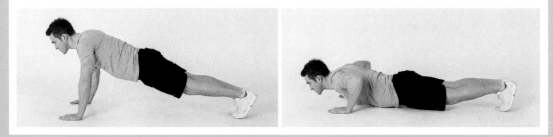

PRESS-UP TO BREAKDANCER

» Perform a prees-up as above, then pivot onto your left arm and leg, letting your other leg and hand come up off the floor. The leg off the floor comes out in front of you. Return to the press-up position, but immediately pivot onto your right hand and right leg.

» Repeat as smoothly as possible.

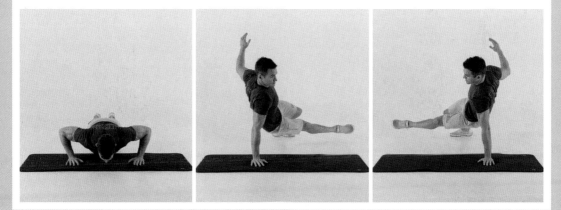

PRONE DUMBBELL PULL-OVER

» Lie flat on a bench, holding a dumbbell vertical in both hands above your chest. Your hands should be under the end of the dumbbell, not holding it by the handle.

» Keep your arms straight and slowly lower the weight in an arc behind your head.

» Pull the weight back up to the starting position and repeat as required.

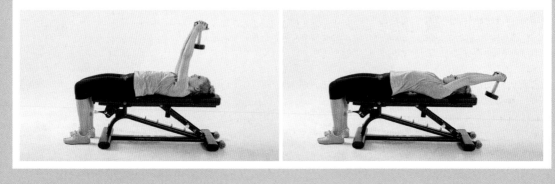

PRONE ROW

» For this exercise, you might need to put the bench on a couple of boxes so that you can stretch your arms out fully and thus get the full range of movement at your disposal. Some gyms have a specific prone row bench, which is much taller than other benches and can be used with a barbell, kettlebells or dumbbells. In the photos we have used a bench without blocks to show the simplest way of performing the excercise.

» Lie on a flat bench face down, holding a barbell or dumbbell or kettlebell in each hand.

» Slowly row the barbell or dumbbells up, engaging your back muscles, then slowly lower at the designated tempo.

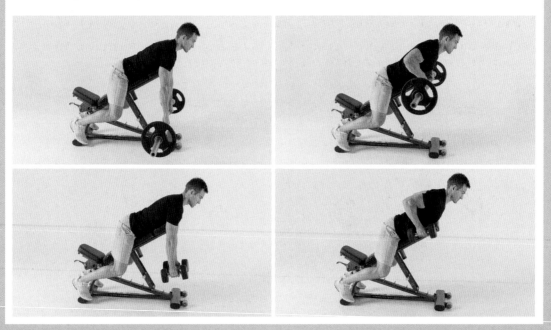

REVERSE LUNGE

» This movement can be done completely on one side before switching, or can be performed in an alternating fashion.

» Stand with your hands on your hips or hanging at your sides. Look directly forward, keeping your chest up and your feet shoulder width apart.

» Take a step to the rear, allowing your hips and knees to flex to lower your body. Contacting the back leg through only the ball of the foot, descend until your knee nearly touches the ground. Use a slow and controlled motion, paying special attention to proper mechanics and posture. The knee should stay in line with the foot, and the thoracic spine should remain neutral. Make sure you weight goes straight down.

» After a brief pause, return to the starting position by driving through the heel of the front leg to extend the knees and hips.

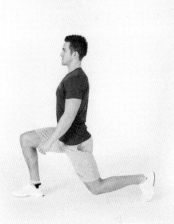

ROMANIAN DEADLIFT

» Pick the bar off the floor using the deadlift technique on page 115. Hold the bar at hip level with a pronated (palms facing down) grip or an alternative grip as shown in the photos. Your shoulders should be back, your back arched, and your knees slightly bent.

» Lower the bar by moving your butt back as far as you can. Keep the bar close to your body, your head looking forward and your shoulders back. Done correctly, you should reach the maximum range of your hamstring flexibility just below the knee. Any further movement will be compensation and should be avoided for this movement. You will have a slight bend in your knees when you are lowering. Make sure to keep your back flat and your head neautral.

» At the bottom of your range of motion, return to the starting position by driving the hips forward to stand up tall. You should feel an increase in tension in your glutes.

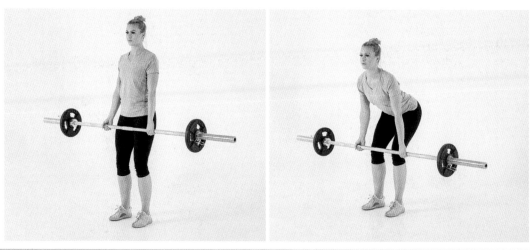

ROTATIONAL CHOP

» Adopt an athletic position with your feet shoulder width apart and your knees slightly bent. Clasp your hands together and hold them out in front of you with fingers interlocked.

» Swing your arms explosively to the left-hand side. You should feel the tension in your abdominals.

» From here, complete a 180-degree swing so that your arms extend out to your right-hand side. Maintain tension in your abdominals.

» Continue to swing from side to side, your feet can rotate as you move and maintaining full control at all times.

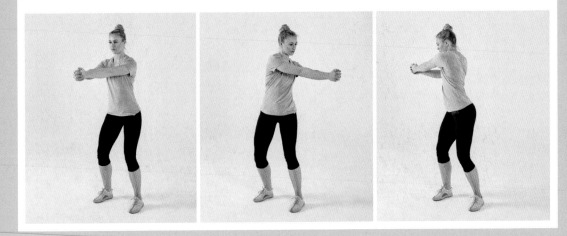

ROWING MACHINE

» Row for the alloted time, making sure to drive with your legs.

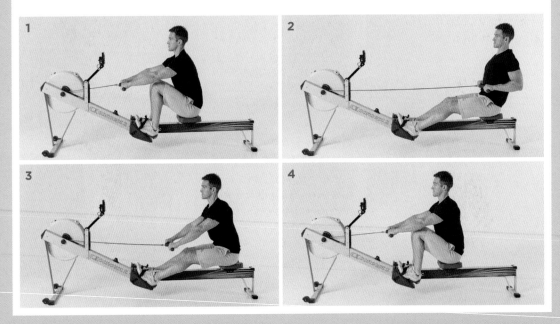

RUNNING ON AND OFF A LOW BOX

» Position a low box in front of you below knee height.

» Step up onto the box with your left leg, then follow with your right leg so that both feet are on the box.

» Step back down onto your left leg. then follow with your right leg.

» Repeat this process of running on and off the box at a high tempo.

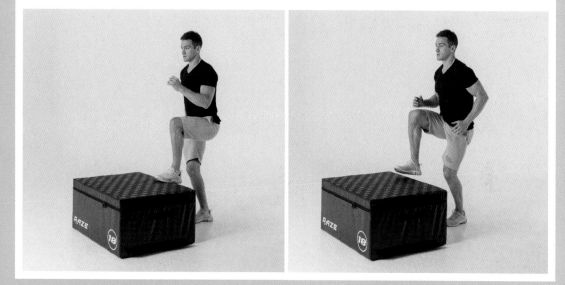

RUNNING ON THE SPOT

» Start with feet slightly apart and run on the spot at a high tempo.

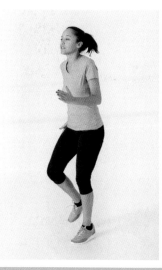

RUNNING ON THE SPOT WITH BUTT KICKS

» This exercise is often called a heel flick, and is something you will have done many times if you are following my prescribed warm-up.

» Standing with feet shoulder width apart, start running on the spot.

» Take a slight lean forward, then try to kick your own backside with each heel in turn. You will feel this in your quads and hip flexors.

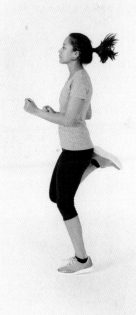

RUNNING ON THE SPOT WITH BURPEES

» Run on the spot and every 5 seconds drop down into a burpee, then jump back up again.

» Run on the spot.

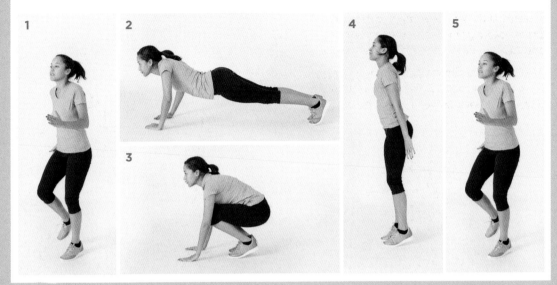

RUNNING ON THE SPOT WITH DOWN AND UPS

» Run on the spot and every 5 seconds go down to the floor in a press-up, letting your chest hit the ground.

» Get up again as quickly as possible, and repeat as required.

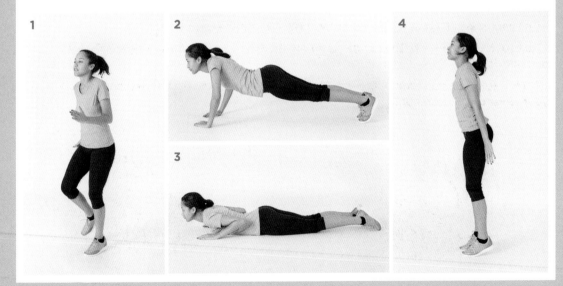

RUNNING ON THE SPOT WITH HIGH KNEES

» This exercise can be performed while running in place or moving over a distance.

» Stand with your feet hip width apart. Drive your right knee towards your chest and quickly place it back on the ground.

» Follow immediately by driving your left knee towards your chest. Continue to alternate knees as quickly as you can.

RUNNING ON THE SPOT WITH TUCK JUMPS

» Run on the spot and every 10 steps, jump your knees up to your chest.

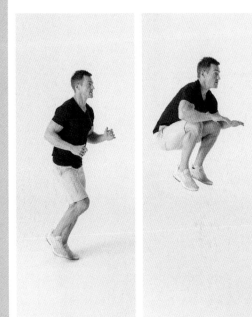

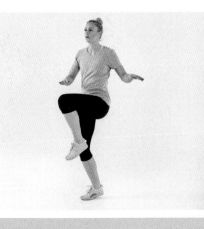

RUSSIAN TWIST

» Lie on your back on the floor, knees up and feet flat on the ground.

» Roll your knees to your left, keeping your left foot on the floor.

» Roll your knees back to the middle, then roll them to the right, keeping the right foot on the floor.

» Do this for the suggested number of reps, trying to go further each time, and feel your lower back loosen off.

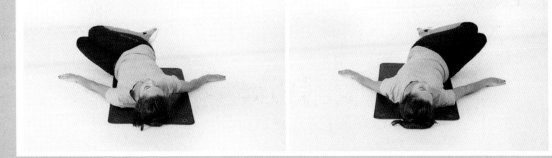

SEAL JACK

» Stand with your feet shoulder width apart and your arms out in front of you. Jump your legs out and spread your arms wide, as though preparing for an exaggerated handclap.

» Jump your feet and arms back in again, clapping your hands together in front of you, arms fully extended. You will look like a seal clapping, hence the name of the exercise.

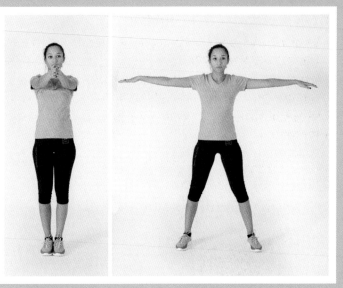

SEATED HAMMER CURL

» Sit on a bench with a straight back. Using a neutral grip, hold two dumbbells by your side, your palms facing inwards and arms fully extended.

» Keeping your palms facing inwards, raise the dumbbells while contracting the biceps until the weights reach shoulder level. At this point the plates of the dumbbells should be facing the ceiling and your palms still facing inwards.

» Lower the weight with a 2-second eccentric (lowering) phase to the starting position.

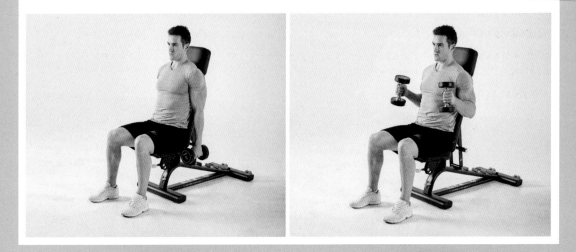

SEATED LATERAL RAISE

» Sit on a bench set at a 90-degree angle. Keeping your back straight, hold two light dumbbells by your sides.

» Keeping your arms straight, lift the dumbbells out to the side until they are level with your face. You should feel the tension in the sides of your shoulders and traps.

» Hold at the top of this movement for 1 second, then lower to the starting position with control.

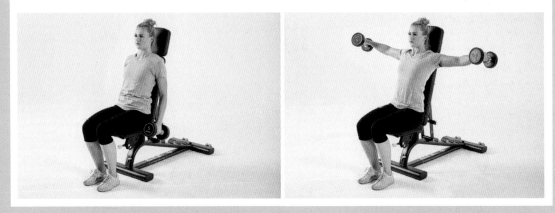

SEATED SHOULDER PRESS

This exercise is performed while sitting on a bench that has back support.

» Place the dumbbells upright on top of your thighs, then raise them one at a time to shoulder height, using your thighs to help propel them into position. Make sure to rotate your wrists so that the palms of your hands are facing forward.

» Exhale and push the dumbbells upward until they touch at the top.

» After a brief pause at the top contracted position, slowly lower the weights to the starting position while inhaling.

» Repeat as required.

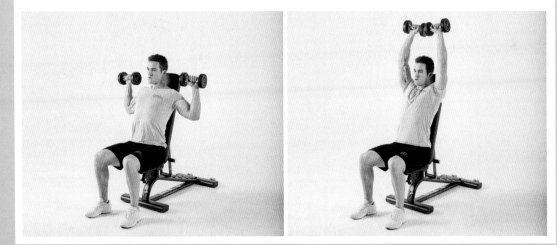

SHOULDER PRESS

» Standing with your feet shoulder width apart, take a dumbbell in each hand. Raise them to head height, with the elbows out at about 90 degrees.

» Maintaining strict technique, with no leg drive or leaning back, extend through the elbow to raise the weights together directly above your head.

» Pause, then slowly return the weight to the starting position.

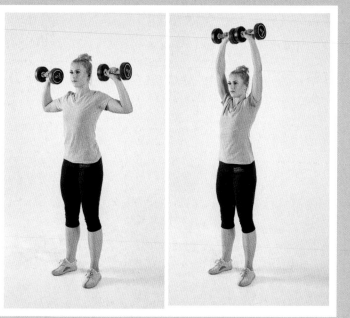

SIDE-LYING OPENS

» Adopt a press-up position with your hands placed in line with your chest, your back straight, your abs tight and your weight distributed evenly between your hands and feet.

» Slowly lift your right hand off the floor and transfer your body weight to your left hand. Move your right arm out to the side and then up towards the ceiling, opening out your chest and engaging your core as you do so. As you do this your right foot will come off the floor and rest on your left foot, so your whole bodyweight is balanced on your left hand and foot.

» At the top of this position your left arm should be pointing towards the ceiling and your body in a T-shape.

» Come back down to the starting position and repeat the process on the other side. Ensure you perform the same number of reps on both sides.

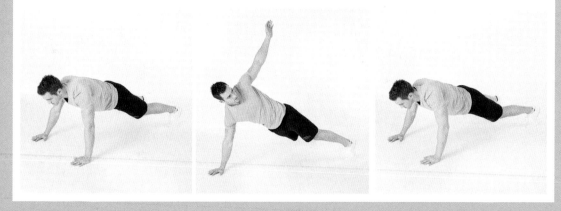

SIDE PLANK HOLD

» Start in a press-up position, then rotate so that you are resting on one hand and your legs are on top of each other. You need to engage you abs, glutes and obliques, and make sure your body doesn't sag in the middle. Do one working set.

» Swap to the other side for the next working set.

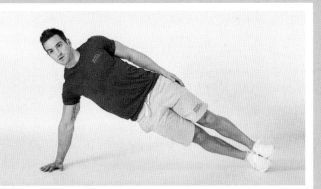

SIDE-TO-SIDE HOP

» Stand in an athletic position, with your feet shoulder width apart. Jump both feet to the left, then immediately to the right.

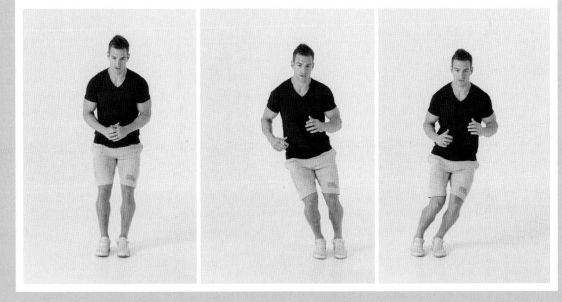

SIDE-TO-SIDE SHUFFLE

» Adopt an athletic position with you feet slightly wider than shoulder width apart, your knees slightly bent and your arms bent at the elbow.

» Shuffle yourfeet to the left, gtaking 10 very fast small steps. Focus on being explosive.

» Repeat the process to the right. Continue alternating left and right.

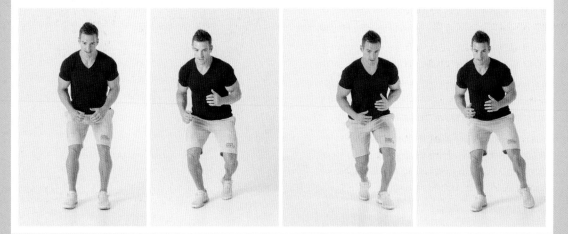

SINGLE-ARM DUMBBELL ROW

» Rest your right hand on a secure bench or platform and hold a dumbbell in your left hand. Bend over the bench so that your back is straight and your weight held securely on your left hand. You will have a bend in your knees and weight through the balls of your feet.

» Row the dumbbell up towards your chest, focusing on squeezing your lat as you do so.

» Lower the dumbbell with control, then repeat as required.

» Repeat the same number of reps on your left side, then rest.

» You can also perform this exercise with one knee and one hand on a bench to balance yourself. You then have a foot out to balance you on the floor. Keeping your back flat, row the dumbbell from the floor.

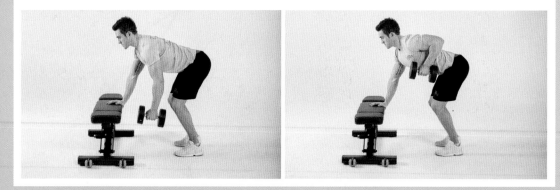

SKATER JUMP

» Stand in an athletic position with your feet shoulder width apart and your knees slightly bent.

» Cross your left leg behind your right leg and bend at the knees into a half squat.

» Push off with your right foot and jump up and across to the left as far as you can.

» Land lightly on your left foot, crossing your right leg behind your left.

» Lower into a half squat, then jump up and across to where you came from as quickly and as powerfully as you can.

» It's really important in this exercise to be balanced when you land, so concentrate fully on using your glutes to explode into the jump.

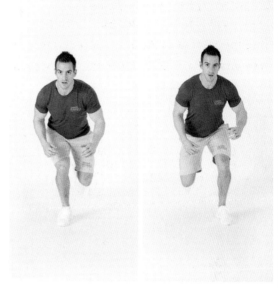

SKIER SWING

» Stand in an athletic position with your feet shoulder width apart, knees slightly bent and arms beside your thighs.

» Lift your arms out to 90 degrees, then bend them at the elbow and swing them backwards so that they straighten behind you. (Imagine a skier using the poles to propel themselves forwards.) Push your hips and hamstrings back as you do this and bend at the trunk.

» Bring your arms forward and straighten back to the athletic position as you do so. Maintain a fluid swinging motion as you perform this exercise.

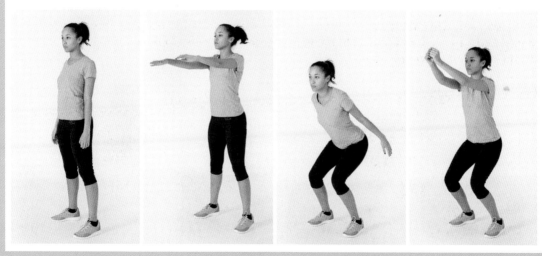

SKIPPING ON THE SPOT WITH A ROPE

» If using a skipping rope, make sure you find a good one that is long enough for your height. There is nothing worse than trying to skip with the wrong length of rope that keeps catching. The best kind of rope will be down to your personal preference. I prefer a heavy one.

» Stand in a good upright stance with the knees relaxed. Your legs don't have to be actually bent, but they should not be locked straight.

» Hold the rope in your hands around waist height.

» Rise up on the balls of your feet, as though standing on tiptoe, then begin jumping up and with both feet together, turning the rope as you do so.

» Skip at full capacity for the required time.

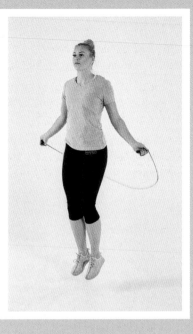

SKIPPING ON THE SPOT WITHOUT A ROPE

» Stand in a good upright stance with the knees relaxed. Your legs don't have to be actually bent, but they should not be locked straight.

» Hold your hands about waist height, with your palms up, as though holding a skipping rope.

» Rise up on the balls of your feet, then begin gently bouncing up and down on both feet.

» Skip at full capacity for the required time.

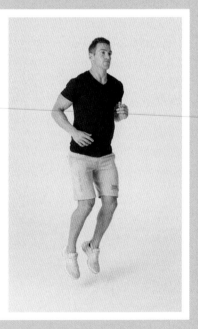

SPEED WALK-OUT PRESS-UP

» Try to do this exercise as dynamically as possible while staying rigid through your torso. You don't want to be rocking about too much as you move.

» Standing tall, bend over slowly and walk your hands out in front of you until you are in a press-up position, your arms slightly extended in front of you, your back straight and your abdominals tight.

» Perform a press-up, then slowly walk your hands back towards your feet until you are standing tall again. You will feel tension through your hamstrings as you walk back up, and might need to bend your legs slightly.

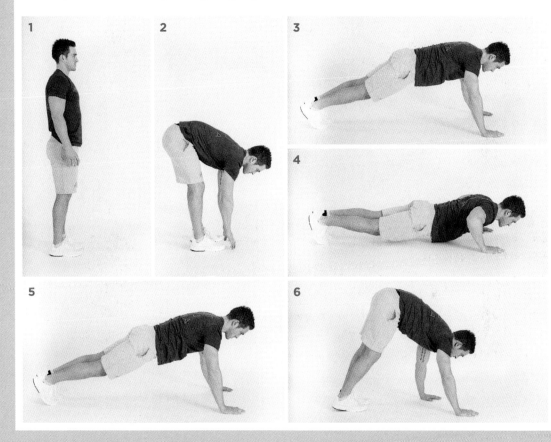

SPIDERMAN MOUNTAIN CLIMBER

» If you have limited mobility, do basic mountain climbers instead of this exercise.

» Start in a normal press-up position, with the weight through your hands and toes.

» Jump your left leg to the outside of your left hand, keeping the right leg in place.

» As you jump the left leg back, jump the right leg to the outside of your right hand.

» This exercise can also be performed with narrow hand placement, i.e. with hands placed closer together than usual.

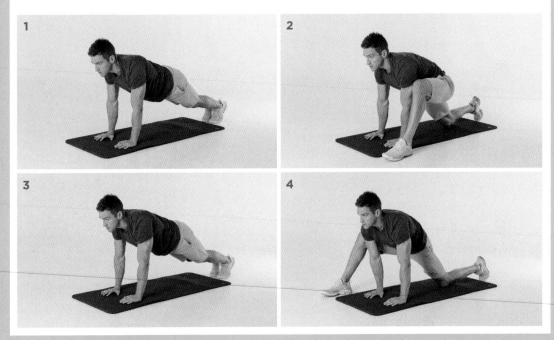

SPIN BIKE OR WATTBIKE RIDE

» Make sure the seat and handlebars are at the correct height; you should be able to fully extend your legs. Also ensure the resistance is set to make the ride hard. On the Wattbike there are two resistance settings – air and magnetic – to create the feel of a real ride.

» Pedal a stationary exercise bike as fast as you can for the specified time.

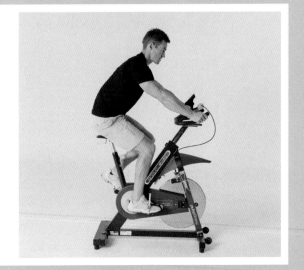

SQUAT JUMP

» Do a basic bodyweight squat. At the bottom of the squat, explode back upwards into a jump so that your whole body is straight and your feet leave the floor.

» As your feet return to the floor, drop back into the squat position and repeat the movement.

» Even though you are doing this dynamically, you need to maintain control the whole time.

» It's hard to maintain control when doing squat jumps, so make sure you stay steady and have good form. Do not allow your back to curve or the weight to come onto your toes when performing these jumps.

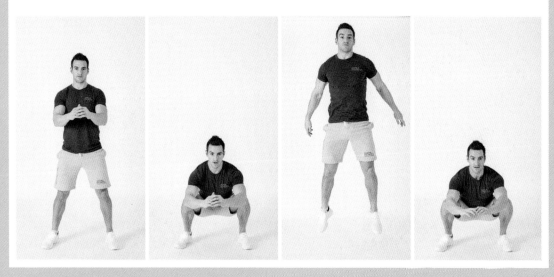

SQUAT TO A BOX, THEN JUMP

» Position a sturdy box or gym bench behind you so that it just touches your bottom when you squat.

» When your bottom touches the box, dynamically jump back up to standing and repeat.

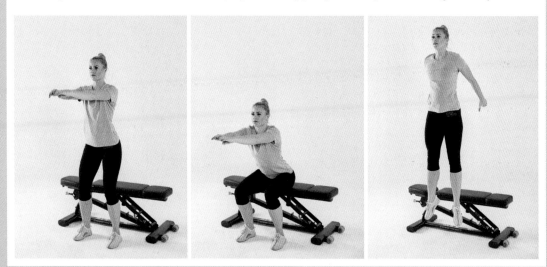

STAR JUMP

» Start with your feet together and arms straight down by your sides.

» Jump your legs apart and raise your arms above your head in a V-shape.

» Jump your legs back in and lower your arms.

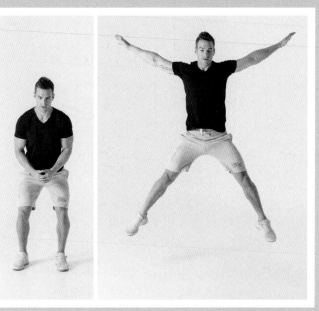

STRAIGHT-LEG ABDOMINAL FLUTTER

» Lie flat on your back on the floor, placing your hands under your bottom or by your sides, palms facing down.

» Raise your legs off the floor by 10cm and flutter them up and down in small movements. Don't take them too high or let them touch the ground during the working set.

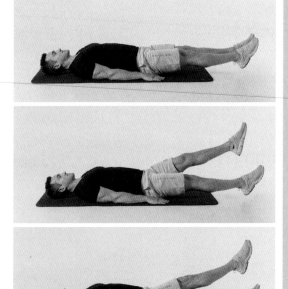

SUMO SQUAT

» Stand with your feet at least at least a metre apart – significantly wider than hip distance.

» Turn your toes out 45 degrees and hold your hands by your sides.

» Lower yourself down by bending your knees, meanwhile raising your hands to meet under your chin. Keep your abs tight and your back straight, and do not let your knees move past your toes when lowering.

» Once your thighs are parallel the floor, drive upwards until your knees are straight and you return to the starting position. Repeat as required.

» It's really important to keep your knees tracking out when doing these squats. Keep your weight through your heels at all times.

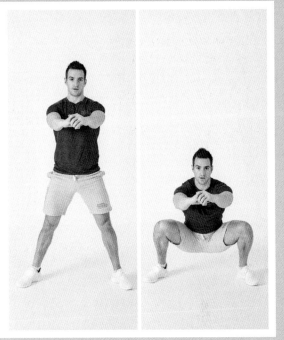

SWISS BALL HAMSTRING PULL

» This exercise will take some practice to get used to. You can put your arms out to the side to balance yourself. The more you dig your heels into the Swiss ball, the more control you have.

» Lie flat on your back with your feet resting on the Swiss ball. You can have your arms out to the side for balance.

» Bridge up on the ball, putting the weight through your heels and driving your hips up.

» Using your heels, roll the ball towards your bottom, driving your hips up higher. Focus on maintaining tension in your hamstrings and glutes at all times.

» Slowly roll the ball back to the start position and repeat as required.

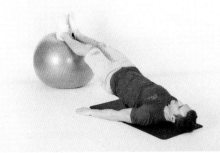
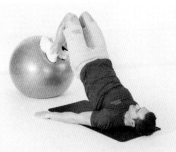

TRAP BAR DEADLIFT

» For this exercise load a trap bar, also known as a hex bar, to an appropriate weight resting on the ground. Stand in the centre of the apparatus and grasp both handles.

» Lower your hips, look forward with your head and keep your chest up.

» Begin the movement by driving through the heels and extend your hips and knees. Avoid rounding your back at all times. You are using your hamstrings and glutes to power you back up.

» When you reach the top of the movement, make sure you engage your glutes.

» At the completion of the movement, lower the weight back to the ground under control.

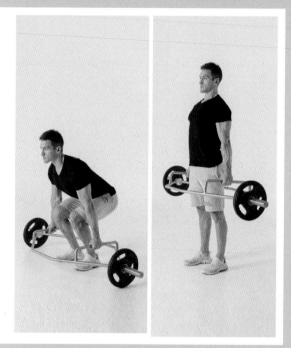

TREADMILL RUN

» In this exercise, make sure you have warmed up properly and understand what speed you are running at. Don't just crank up the machine and jump onto it.

» Put your feet either side of a treadmill and set the speed to the highest setting you can manage for the allotted time. Wait for it to reach that speed.

» Hold onto the handrails as you jump on the treadmill and find your stride. Let go of the handrails and run for the allotted time.

» Once the time is up, jump off the machine with your feet to the side. Rest there, then jump back on for the next rep.

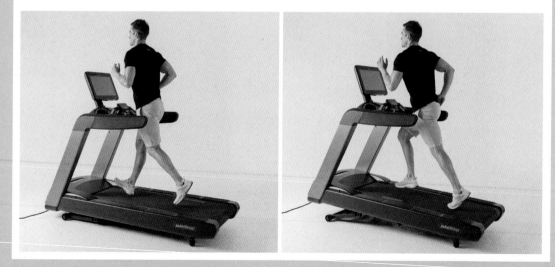

TRICEP ROPE PUSH-DOWN

» Position the cable on a cable-pull machine at chest height and secure a rope grip.

» Hold onto the rope and push downwards until your elbows are straight and your arms fully extended. Concentrate on engaging your triceps as you perform this movement.

» At the bottom of the movement, pull the rope slightly outwards. Return to the starting position with control and repeat. If necessary, you can put one foot in front of the other to balance yourself.

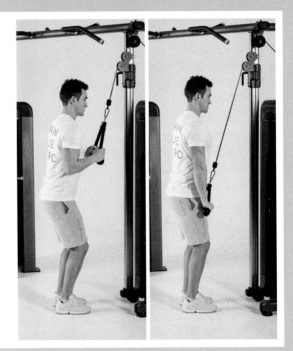

TUCK JUMP

» Stand with your feet shoulder width apart, knees slightly bent and arms by your sides.

» Push up explosively, bringing both knees up to your chest. Land normally and repeat as required.

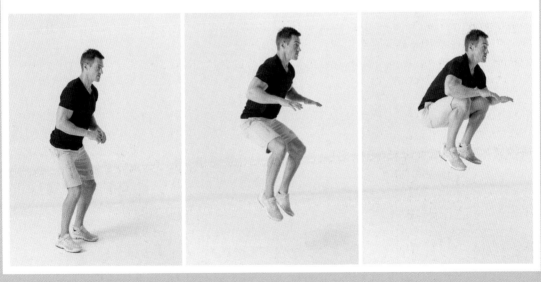

WALKING LUNGE

» Stand with your feet shoulder width apart and go into a forward lunge. Do not allow your front knee to travel forward over your toes. Imagine you have a weighted cable that runs through your body, pulling you down rather than forward.

» Push your weight through the outstretched foot, then drive your other leg through so that you go back to standing. You then lunge out with the other leg in the same way. You are doing this in a dynamic way, moving forward each time you lunge out.

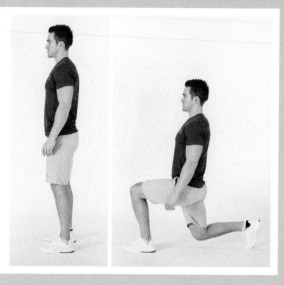

WALL PRESS-UP

» Keeping your arms straight, place your hands shoulder width apart against a wall.

» Slowly lower your face towards the wall, getting as close as you can without actually touching it. The further back you set your feet, the harder it is.

» Push out again, then repeat as required.

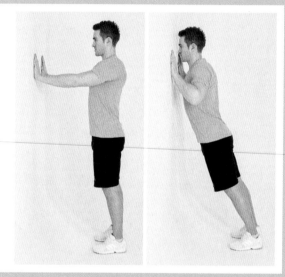

WEIGHTED GLUTE BRIDGE

» Lie on your back with your feet on the floor with you knees bent, pointing towards the ceiling and a barbell on your pelvis. You might wish to use a pad to prevent the barbell from digging into your hips.

» Keeoing your weight in your heels, drive your hips upwards, contracting your glutes as you do so. Drive until your back is straight and hips are level with your knees, drive the weight up along with your hips. Take a slight pause at the top and control the weight on the way down.

See pictures opposite » » »

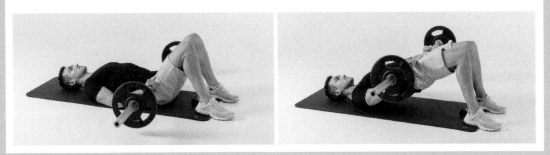

WIDE HAND PLACEMENT PRESS-UPS

» Hold yourself in a front plank position, with your hands wider than shoulder width apart, and level with your chest.

» Lower yourself down as far as possible without touching the floor. Drive back to the starting position and repeat.

» Imagine pushing your hands together while doing the press-up to engage your chest muscles

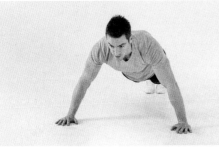

WIDE WALL PRESS-UPS

» Keeping your arms straight, place your hands wider than shoulder width apart against a wall.

» Slowly lower your face towards the wall, getting as close as you can without actually touching it. The further back you set your feet, the harder it is.

» Push out again, then repeat as required.

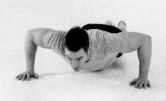

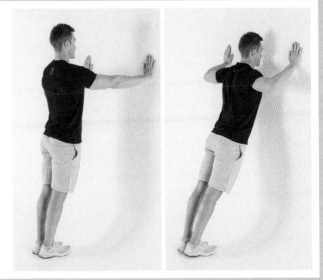

LISS MENU

Here is a selection of low-intensity steady state (LISS) cardio sessions that you can use on your days off if you want to do extra training. They can be done using any standard cardio equipment you find in a gym, or you can just use your own body. In a basic LISS session, you should aim to work for 30–45 minutes so that you are sweating and challenging yourself throughout the workout. However, you need to be able to complete the full session, so don't set too fast a pace for yourself. LISS is not HIIT, so you are not working to your maximum. It's about working for the duration of the session.

TRAINING WITH EQUIPMENT

Cardio machines are really simple to use, but do make sure you get everything set up correctly before you start. Here are some pointers:

Cross-trainer

Turn up the resistance, as this machine is far too easy without any.

Rowing machine

Make sure your feet are strapped in and that you maintain good posture.

Running machine

Always add a little incline; 1–2% is good.

Spin bike

Make sure you have the seat and handlebars set to the correct height. You also need to ride against some resistance to make the ride hard.

Stepper/Stairmaster

A set of revolving steps that can be set to different levels of fitness. It's good for cardio workouts and lower body conditioning and is excellent for burning fat.

VersaClimber

This is my favourite piece of cardio equipment for doing hard, sharp blasts of exercise, but it can be great for LISS as well. It mimics the way you climb up something vertically, and is far and away the best for full body conditioning. There are loads of ways to use it, but simply choosing a famous monument to climb is great. The image is shown on a screen and charts your way up it. However, I find the best way to get through a workout longer than 30–45 minutes on this piece of equimpent is to do 40 seconds of long strides and 20 seconds of short strides. If you are using it for HIIT work, you want long fast strides done as quickly as possible. You do have the option to add or take away resistance. I always do it wIth no resistance so that I'm working with my own bodyweight.

Wattbike

Make sure the seat and handlebars are at the correct height; you should be able to fully extend your legs. Also ensure the resistance is set to make the ride hard. On the Wattbike there are two resistance settings – air and magnetic – to create the feel of a real rIde.

TRAINING WITHOUT EQUIPMENT

If you don't fancy using cardio equipment in the gym, there
are other ways to get your LISS training done.

Take the dog for a 30–40 minute walk or jog

This is really easy and provides good steady-state cardio. Setting a brisk pace will ensure you actually get some physical benefit. Also, the faster you walk a dog on a lead, the more it concentrates on walking as opposed to sniffing and investigating everything around it, a tip I learnt from TV's 'dog whisperer' Cesar Millan. If you feel more adventurous, you could also take the dog for a run.

Ride a bike for 30–60 minutes

This provides a good steady-state workout, and you don't have to be Sir Bradley Wiggins to get the benefit. A ride is great if you want to de-stress in the evening after work, but if you are super-keen, why not use the bike for your commute to and from work? If you have kids, going out together for a bike ride is a great way to get them exercising.

You can of course ride your bike to the gym, which will get you warmed up for your session and reduce the time you need to warm up when you get there.

Your bike rides should always be at a steady pace, and energetic enough to build up a light sweat by the end. You can of course use a fixed bike at home or in the gym if you prefer.

Jog or run at a steady pace for 30–45 minutes

I would suggest you run on grass rather than a hard surface as it's easier on your joints, but if you have to go road running, make sure you choose some good footwear. You need good supportive shoes or you will develop all sorts of issues further down the line.

You can run to the gym or to work if it's not miles away. Just ensure it's far enough to work up a sweat. Again, this will be a good warm-up before your actual training session. However, if it's too far or very hard going, it will detract from your actual gym session, which is never good.

There are loads of smart watches and fittech available that can track your heart rate and how far you run. It's not essential to use one, but it's always good to collect data so that you can add it to your training notes. You will then be able to adjust your run each week, adding or reducing time and distance, depending on how you feel.

Go for a swim

This is another way to get your steady-state work done. It makes a change from working on cardio equipment, but I must admit that I find swimming lengths super-boring. For this reason, I like to break it up with a combination of jogging, hopping, squat jumps and underwater swimming. If you want to do the same, I suggest you jog up and down the pool for a couple of lengths, perform some bodyweight work, such as press-ups and crunches, outside the pool, or do some bodyweight work, such as calf raises, squats and jumps, in the pool, then go into a few full lengths doing whatever stroke you want. After that, you could do some underwater swimming, which really pushes your lung capacity and tests your fitness level. Start by doing, say, 8 strokes underwater, then surface for a breath and go back under to finish the length. As you are not doing a flat-out conditioning session, you can take more rest after doing this. Complete 5 sets, then move back to bodyweight work or traditional lengths.

Chapter 5
RECOVERY

Whether you are a seasoned pro or a complete novice in the world of training, recovery will play a huge role in getting you through my programme. It will also help you to continue training long after you have completed the basic 8 week plan or the more extensive 12 week plan.

As a rugby player, I'm aware that the game puts a huge strain on the body, the equivalent of being involved in a car crash. I therefore take recovery very seriously because I have only 6–7 days between games to get myself back to full fitness.

I am always striving for the best ways to recover from muscle soreness, tiredness and overtraining. **The one thing I know for sure is that there is no magic bullet**. Instead, it's a combination of different things that helps me to feel better – mainly massage, the use of an electronic muscle stimulator called a compex, sleep and banded mobility work. However, that combination will be different for each and every one of you reading this book.

If you are training hard enough, you are going to suffer from DOMS – Delayed Onset Muscle Soreness – which means that a day or two after training you will be walking like John Wayne and wondering what the hell you have done to yourself. There will also be times when you are injured – it happens to all of us.

Recovery does not mean simply sitting on your bottom or lying in bed. Don't get me wrong: rest and sleep play a big part in getting back to normal and at times they're the best things you can do, but they're far from being the whole story. **What's really needed is an active approach**.

First, if you have real injury concerns, you need to see a doctor, or at least a physiotherapist. I'm not in favour of training through injuries as a badge of toughness. This habit has always been around, especially in professional sport, but has grown since the advent of things like CrossFit and other training modalities, a programme of gruelling workouts that can be done at home or in a 'box' (a gym with minimal equipment but all very specific to that genre of training). I'm not against CrossFit – it has a lot to offer – but I don't think its culture is helpful to amateurs. The gruelling sessions and lack of technique mean that people are more susceptible to injury, but they grin and bear it as they don't want to let the team down. This is obviously not unique to CrossFit, I am merely using it as an example of training where this is more prevalent.

Training hurt is not a clever thing to do, though I can understand it if, say, the world championships are at stake, or you have a world cup final the next day. In that case, I'm all for cracking on as long as your performance will not jeopardise the team. What does seem mad to me is muddling through a Tuesday evening workout just because you want to look tough.

Injuries are a fact of training and need to be looked after properly so that you can return to action straight away. Please see my tips opposite.

SUGGESTED RECOVERY AND INJURY PROTOCOLS

Remember the mnemonic **RICE** – Rest, Ice, Compression and Elevation – because these are the key things to do with any injury in the first instance.

» **Rest the injury** after it occurs, and stop training.

» **Ice** any strained, bruised or very sore areas for 15–20 minutes maximum every couple of hours. Remember, it's not about trying to freeze yourself.

» **Compress** the injury with a compression bandage (available from most chemists) to reduce swelling. There is also the option of renting or purchasing a Game Ready machine, which ices and compresses at the same time. These are expensive, but worth it if you are a sportsperson or used to regular injury.

» **Elevate** the injury on a raised surface, ideally higher than your heart. This will help to reduce swelling.

» **Take hot and cold contrast baths.** Spend 1 minute in each, finishing in a hot bath. Alternatively, use a cold bath and a hot shower, or simply hot and cold showers. I find this regime works well after heavy training sessions, and I much prefer it to straight ice baths. A lot of lads swear that 10-minute ice baths work wonders, but I hate them and can never last that long. Please note that straight ice baths are best avoided after leg weight sessions as some research indicates that they can limit results. Like most things in the fitness and health world there are conflicting studies that both promote and denounce ice baths. It all comes down to what works for you individually.

» **Add some magnesium or Epsom salts to your bath water.** They replenish the magnesium your muscles have lost, so a good hot soak is not only relaxing, but maximises recovery. Use these salts after a heavy session, but never within 48 hours of an upcoming game or performance because they can dehydrate you and might also make you feel slightly heavy legged.

» **Get a massage from a qualified masseur.** The Sports Massage Institute (www.thesma. org) is a good place to look. Sometimes a few sessions of soft tissue massage can cure tight areas and prevent injury further down the line. You should look to add these in once a week.

» **Try wearing compression garments.** These are believed to improve bloodflow, thus removing lactic acid. Some manufacturers also suggest wearing them during sport to improve power and endurance. I haven't come across much scientific evidence to support their use, but the placebo effect is well known, so if you find them helpful, feel free to use them. The improvement may be tiny, but look what Dave Brailsford, the British cycling mastermind, achieved by accumulating marginal gains. Once you've nailed diet and training, picking up little improvements in the area of recovery can be really significant, especially if you combine the recovery protocols. Pick up 1 per cent from each one and that's 5 per cent improvement across the board, which is huge.

>> **Buy an electronic muscle stimulator (EMS).** Sometimes known as a Compex, one of the brands available, this device has many functions that can help with recovery. It's great for rebuilding wasted muscle after operations, but also has some very nifty massage functions. Whenever I have bad DOMS or tight muscles, I put the electrodes on the affected area and it works really well. Also, if you have any problem muscles that don't fire very well because of pain, using an EMS device on it as a warm-up is very effective. However, don't go too mad when using the machine as it can increase DOMS tenfold.

>> **Get into yoga or Pilates.** I have tried both in a limited fashion and found results in terms of mobility. And let me tell you, yoga is no soft option for those with limited mobility. I used to do one-on-one yoga sessions and I would be sweating within 30 seconds of starting. I honestly reckon that if I didn't play sport and had more time to dedicate to yoga, I would get more value from it, but I stopped as it was tiring me out and the results were limited. However, I'm sure some of you will love it and find it to be a game changer.

You should be careful about Bikram yoga. This is done in a very hot room, the idea being that the warmer your core temperature, the more supple you become. However, it can massively dehydrate you and put your muscles under stress. It's great in your down time, but if you are looking to lift heavy and train hard, you don't need any added complications.

>> **Warm up and recover properly.** Getting both right will help you to avoid issues down the line. Essentially, you are more dynamic when warming up and can be a little more static when recovering. I actually do stretching exercises for mobility throughout my lifting sessions, and take rest periods in between HIIT work. Of course, if you're doing a flat-out conditioning session, you probably won't have the energy to stretch and mobilise.

>> **Keep hydrated throughout the day.** When playing for England, we rugby players weigh ourselves pre- and post-match to see how much weight we have lost through sweating. I often lose 2–3kg during a game, which can hugely affect how the body performs, so balance needs to be restored. If you don't get yourself back to where you started, it can adversely affect your recovery and this in turn will affect your training. The message is simple: keep up your water intake throughout the day and post-training. Even if you think you are drinking enough, drink more.

>> **Eat well.** You should be doing this anyway because diet affects every aspect of your physical and mental health, but getting your nutrition right is also one of the biggest factors in recovery. Of course you need to fuel what you are doing, but equally important is to replenish what you have exhausted. Whatever your goal, this training programme is demanding, so it's important that you don't neglect your diet in any way.

>> **Sleep and nap soundly.** Good rest is the biggest tool in recovery, which is why I talk about it in detail on page 187. If you are getting only five hours a night, it's not enough, and could be having negative effects on every aspect of your well-being. Even worse, in terms of this programme, you could be inhibiting the changes you are trying to get from your body.

MOBILITY

Contrary to what you might think by looking at me, I spend very little time trying to put on muscle or working out in the gym. Mobility is my focus, something that I think about every day and plan most of my sessions around. However, mobility sessions as most people know them involve long-hold static stretching, and I hate stretching with a passion. Perhaps it's because I never feel a discernible difference, or the results don't come quickly enough to capture my attention. Whatever the case, I know the importance of mobility – the England coach puts a huge emphasis on mobile players – so I have spent a long time finding more tolerable ways to achieve it: yoga, partner stretching, foam rolling, you name it.

Ultimately, what came to my rescue was a book called *Becoming a Supple Leopard* by Dr. Kelly Starrett. It teaches correct movement patterns and how to lift properly, but also provides a stretching routine that can be followed straight away. I found it super-easy to understand, and as soon as I started, I began getting results. At last, here was something I enjoyed and could stick with.

I find that doing mobility work between sets of weights, pre-training and post-training makes all the difference to how I function and feel. It certainly limits muscle soreness and makes recovery from tough sessions far quicker. With this in mind, I've devised a mobility circuit that I really like and that I believe will help you. It works from the feet up to the shoulders and can be done on recovery days or during your actual training sessions.

Remember, you are not expected to get everything perfect straight away. I certainly didn't and still don't. It's a progression. When I list certain options, the idea is to start with the simplest and work up to the more complicated as you improve. You are asked to hold each stretch and, as you do so, you can slowly oscillate in and out of tension, and try to find tight angles. Do this for two minutes, then swap legs or move on.

MOBILISING IN THE EARLY DAYS

Foam rolling is a key tool for anyone preparing for training or about to undertake training for the first time. It is also very useful for those returning to training after a prolonged absence. Don't spend hours on this or do it aggressively: 6–8 slow rolls on each muscle area should be enough. Apart from rolling backwards and forwards, it's also good to roll slowly from side to side.

Inevitably, there are many opinions in the fitness world on whether foam rolling does any good. From experience, I know that targeting areas of soreness with a foam roller works well for me, so I imagine it will for you too. Start by targeting the super-tight areas and try to get some release, but don't overdo it; some tissues will never loosen off, and if you do too much, you can end up switching off the very muscles you are about to train with. See foam rolling as a way of self trigger pointing as opposed to trying to 'roll tissues out'.

MOBILISING

UPPER BACK ROLL

LOWER BACK ROLL

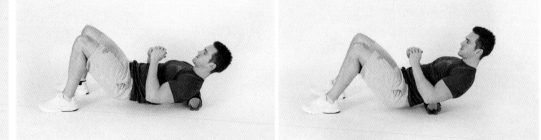

CALVES ROLL

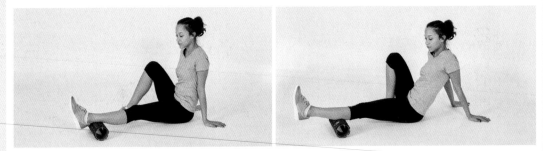

GLUTE ROLL

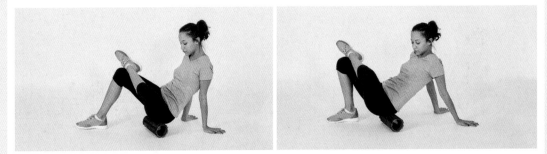

HAMSTRING ROLL

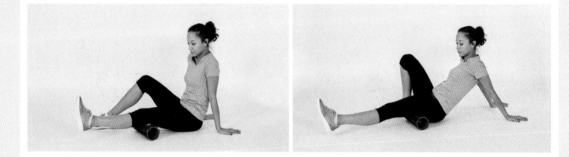

QUAD ROLL

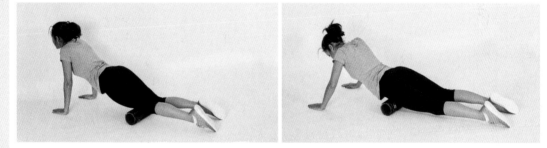

ADUCTORS ROLL

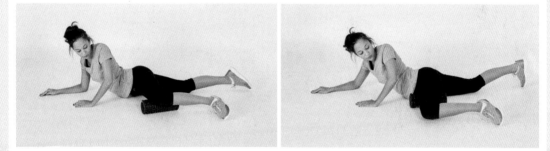

MOBILITY CIRCUIT

The exercises below can be done as a circuit, or can be cherry-picked and used individuallly.

ANKLE MOBILITY:

Put a band around a fixed object, then put a band around the top of your ankle, either facing away from where the band is fixed, or towards it. If you are facing away, have the band sit just just on the front of your ankle in the crease. Put tension through the band and slowly bend your knee over your foot. Do this at different angles to loosen the tissue.

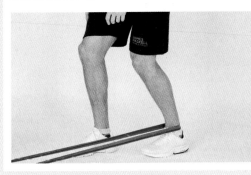

BANDED HIP OPENS:

Hook a gym band around a fixed object, and put the other end around the hip you want to open. Starting on your hands and knees, position your right foot next to your right hand, making sure you keep your right shin vertical. You want the band to pull you to the side or diagonally. Slowly pulse in and out of the stretch, seeking out tight corners. Do this for 2–3 minutes on each hip.

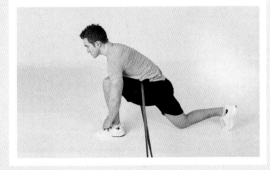

BANDED GLUTE STRETCH:

Hook a gym band around a fixed object and put the other end around the top of your left hip crease. Kneel on the ground and load your weight over your left knee, keeping your femur (thigh) vertical. Swing your left leg across and underneath your body, pinning it in place with your right knee and bodyweight. Keeping the majority of your weight over your left knee, drop your left hip towards the ground. Think about driving the head of your femur through the side of your butt. You will feel tension in your glutes. Hold this position for 2–3 minutes, then swap the band and put your right leg underneath you and repeat.

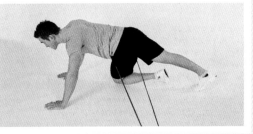

FEET FASCIA ROLLS:

You can do these either seated or standing. Put one of your feet on a tennis ball, hockey ball or golf ball and place enough bodyweight on it to feel tension and slight discomfort. Roll your foot over the ball, sideways, backwards and forwards, finding all the areas of tightness. Do this for 2–3 minutes, or as long as you like, then repeat with the other foot. You can increase the bodyweight on the ball as you improve. After my most recent toe surgery, this exercise has become a staple of my mobility plan.

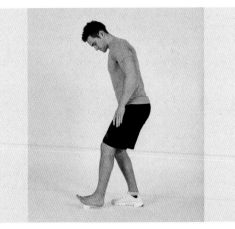

QUAD STRETCH:

Kneel with your back to a wall and your feet just touching it. Slide your left leg back so that your shin is vertical against the wall and your knee is pushed into the right angle at the bottom of the wall. Squeeze your butt to stabilise your lower back, then bring your right foot forward, keeping the shin vertical. If you struggle to get all the way up, you can hold onto a small box or chair in front of you for balance. Still squeezing your left glute, lower your hips towards the ground. Stay in this position for 2–3 minutes and twist your hips from side to side to work through any tight areas. You can then return to a full upright position. Another method is to get into the same position but use a band to stretch.

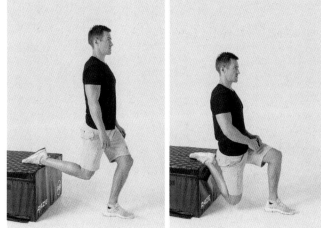

HAMSTRING STRETCH:

Hook a gym band around a fixed object, put the other end around the top of one leg and walk forwards to create tension. It helps if your banded leg is positioned slightly in front of your free leg. Fold forward from your hips, keeping your belly tight and your back flat, and plant your hands on the ground. If you can't reach the ground without rounding your back, position a box or bench in front of you. Straighten your leg and drive your hips back. Still keeping your back as flat as possible, bend your knee. Keeping your weight on your feet, continue to floss backwards and forwards by extending and flexing your knees. Aim to do 20–30 bends.

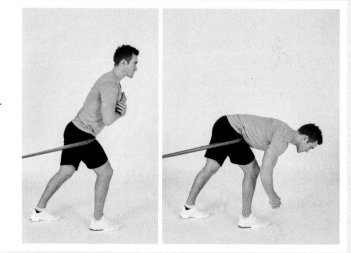

LATERAL STRETCH:

Hook a gym band around a fixed object, put one wrist through the other end and grab both sides of the band in that hand. Use your opposite hand to bias your right arm into external rotation so that your palm is facing up and your thumb is pointing towards the outside of your body. Keep your arm locked in an externally rotated position. Create tension by sinking your hips back and lowering your torso towards the ground. With your arm externally rotated in the overhead position, contract and relax, trying to encourage the shoulder into an increased range of movement. Do this for 2–3 minutes, then repeat on the other side, with the band around your left hand.

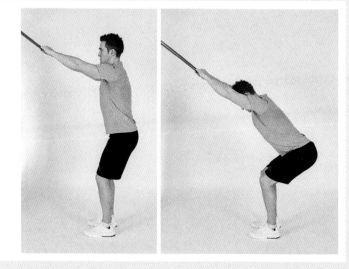

PEC STRETCH:

Hook a gym band around a fixed object and put the other end around your right hand, pulling to create tension. Rotate your palm upwards, favouring external rotation of your shoulder. Keeping your arm externally rotated and your shoulder back, turn away from the band and twist your upper body in a counterclockwise direction. This opens up the chest and arm and hits all the relevant tissues, helping them to loosen. Do this for 2–3 minutes on each side, working out the tight corners, then swap over to the other hand.

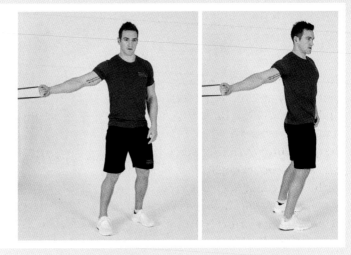

SHOULDER MOBILISATION:

Hook a gym band around a fixed object and put your right hand through the other end. Wind up your right shoulder into extension by turning your body 180 degrees in a counterclockwise direction so that you are facing away from the fixed end of the band. As you step through with your right foot, rotate your right hand so that your palm is positioned towards the ceiling. This helps bias more internal rotation of your arm. With your banded hand exaggerated into extension, you can contract, relax and go hunting for some tight corners by lowering your elevation and twisting your upper body. Do this for 2–3 minutes, then repeat on the other side, with the band around your left hand.

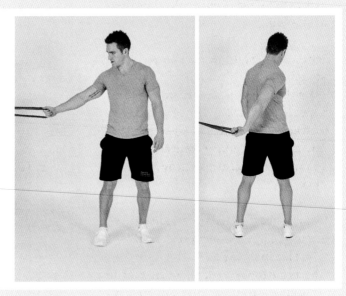

SLEEP

No matter how hard you train or how well you eat, if you don't get good-quality sleep and rest, you will be limiting your results and doing yourself harm. Of course, there are people all over the internet and social media who boast about sleeping only a few hours a night while remaining super-creative. Good on them, I say, but it's not what I recommend or believe in. (I have to be a little careful as my hero The Rock sleeps only four hours a night, or so he says, but I will excuse him this one fault.)

Inadequate rest and recovery can negatively affect muscle repair, put you at greater risk of injury, cause loss of motivation, bring slower results and make you plateau. The ultimate risk, of course, is that you will run out of steam and give up completely.

I know from experience that I cannot operate without 7–8 hours of sleep. If I don't get that amount, I never feel recovered, and it affects me for the next few days. Of course, it's not always possible to get this amount, especially if you have kids. In that case, the most important thing is quality, not quantity.

HOW TO GET THE BEST POSSIBLE SLEEP

There are a few key things that you can do to improve your sleep.

>> **Get a good-quality mattress.** We each spend a third of our life asleep, yet often neglect our sleeping arrangements. Since I started playing professional rugby and good sleep became essential, I have taken more interest in my mattress. For too long I was sleeping on something soft and it meant that I woke up with bad muscle soreness, feeling pretty unrecovered. Eventually, I bit the bullet and invested in a memory foam mattress. The results were pretty clear almost straight away. Within a couple of days I was sleeping so much better and waking up less stiff. The benefits were further proved recently when I moved house and once again found myself sleeping on a dodgy mattress. It caused hell in my lower back. Once again I bought a mattress from ErgoFlex and I was very quickly sleeping far better.

>> **Buy decent pillows.** Finding something suitable has been a big issue for me because 14 years of a contact sport and lifting weights have left me with a very stiff neck. Fortunately, I have it about nailed now, but it was a case of trial and error. Without good supportive pillows, I simply don't sleep, or if I do sleep, I wake up the next morning with a headache. Sleeping with super-soft or lumpy pillows means you will not get the best out of your sleep, so play around with what works for you and don't scrimp, or you will regret it.

>> **Make your bedroom a calm and quiet place.** It should be a zone just for sleep, not for chilling, watching TV or scrolling through your phone. It's all too easy to think you'll just take a quick look at something and then to find that an hour or more has passed. Doing anything that stimulates the mind makes it much harder to get to sleep. You need to mentally link your bedroom with shutting down, not waking up. That means removing any electronic devices such as tvs, laptops and mobile phones, and keeping the room as dark and quiet as possible. Black-out curtains and blinds are a good investment.

>> **Keep the bedroom cool and well oxygenated.** The optimum temperature for sleeping is around 18°C (65°F), but again it's best to experiment to find what suits you. Some research shows that having the window open is a good idea, as sleeping in a cool room will improve the nature of your sleep. There are also studies that show your body burns more calories if it is cold, which is useful if you are trying to lose weight.

>> **Go to bed and get up at a regular time.** I find that going to bed around 10.30pm makes a big difference to how I feel in the morning, especially if I get my preferred 7–8 hours. Similarly, getting up at the same time every day seems to do more good than having a lie-in.

>> **Supplement your sleep if you wish.** My favourite sleep-inducer is ZMA (see page 216). It always helps me have a really deep sleep, but can have the side-effect of giving vivid dreams. I also use a supplement called Amino Man which is a blend of products that help recovery and sleep.

NAPS

I have never been good at napping, but when preparing for the rugby season or going into periods of real physical development, I try to nap in the afternoon for an hour maximum. I know this is not possible for everyone, but getting even 20–30 minutes or so can really boost your performance.

Find a dark, cool and quiet place for your nap, and make sure it's free from distracting technology. (It's a great excuse to get off your phone for a bit.) If you are not used to naps, or you nap for too long, you might feel even more tired after taking a snooze. That's why it's important to nap for no longer than an hour, and to give yourself enough time to wake fully before doing your next thing. I always have an espresso with some coconut oil in it to kickstart me again for the afternoon, whether that is training or working.

NO MATTER HOW HARD YOU TRAIN OR HOW WELL YOU EAT, IF YOU DON'T GET GOOD QUALITY REST YOU WILL BE YOU WILL BE LIMITING YOUR RESULTS.

Chapter 6
NUTRITION

The importance of diet is discussed by all sorts of people in all sorts of contexts. If you follow any of my social media channels or my website, jameshaskell.com, you will know that I often talk about it as the cornerstone of everything you do in relation to taking part in sport or making changes to your body.

Having said that, beginners do not need to worry about too much detail when it comes to nutrition in the early days – they certainly don't need to get bogged down in the detail given later in this chapter. That's why I want to start by outlining in very simple terms what those new to fitness and healthy eating need to do.

NUTRITION FOR BEGINNERS

The first thing you have to decide is if you want to lose fat or gain muscle. In both cases, you need to alter the amount of fuel (calories) you put into your body, so let's look at that next.

CALORIES

A calorie (kcal) is a unit of energy. It refers to both the energy content of food and drink, and the energy we expend during physical activity. For example, a banana might put 86 calories into our body, while a 1-mile walk might use up 100 calories.

About 60–75 per cent of our daily calorie intake is used by the body just to keep itself ticking over while at rest, i.e. the heart beating, the blood circulating, the lungs and brain functioning. This figure is called the Basal Metabolic Rate (BMR). The remaining percentage of our calorie intake is used for physical activity. The more active we are, the more we need to eat, and vice versa.

The total number of calories we need to put into our body is our BMR multiplied by the amount of activity we do to get our Total Daily Energy Expenditure (TDEE), which is explained a bit later.

Whatever your fitness goal, you need to understand two fundamentals about calories. **If you want to lose weight, you need to eat fewer calories. If you want to gain muscle, you have to eat more.** However, it's important to understand that not all calories are created equal. A jam doughnut might well have the same calorie count as a steak, but it would be lunacy to think they have the same nutritional value. Never be fooled into thinking otherwise.

The number of calories it takes to maintain your current shape prior to starting *Perfect Fit* is your BMR multiplied by the amount of specific activity you do daily. This would then give you a figure known as your TDEE. You'll need to do some maths to work these out, but it's easy, believe me. I never understand figures and if there was an easier way I would show you!

HOW TO CALCULATE YOUR EXISTING BMR AND TDEE

You can pay fitness consultants a lot of money to work out these figures for you, or spend a few minutes doing them yourself. Come on – have a go! The two formulas (one for men and the other for women) are given below, and there's an example to show you how they work.

Start by measuring your height in centimetres and weighing yourelf in kilograms. Make a note of these two figures on a piece of paper. Now get your calculator out.

BMR calculation for men
88.362 + (13.397 x weight in kg) + (4.799 x height in cm) – (5.677 x age in years)

BMR calculation for women
447.593 + (9.247 x weight in kg) + (3.098 x height in cm) – (4.330 x age in years)

Example
If we were doing the BMR calculation for me, I would insert my weight, height and age (shown below in **bold**). I'd then do the calculations in each set of brackets, add the first two results to 88.362, and from that figure I'd subtract the last result to arrive at the answer, as follows:

88.362 + (13.397 x **120 kg**) + (4.799 x **193cm**) - (5.677 x **31**) = 2446.222
In other words, 88.362 + 1607.64 + 926.207 – 175.987 = 2446.222

The next step is to find your Total Daily Energy Expenditure – the amount of energy you exert per day.

Calculate your TDEE
First you must decide what level of exercise you have been doing before starting the fitness plan. Look at the list below and be honest!

>> Little or no exercise: x 1.2
>> Light exercise (1–3 days of training per week): x 1.375
>> Moderate exercise (3–5 days per week): x 1.55
>> Heavy exercise (6–7 days per week): x 1.725
>> Very heavy exercise (twice a day or extra heavy workouts): x 1.9

For example, I do five training sessions a week, so I multiply my BMR of 2446 by 1.55 which gives my TDEE of 3791 – the number of calories I need to maintain my current body shape.

Once you want to start the programme, you need to multiply your BMR by 1.55 because in both the 8-week and the 12-week programmes we are asking you to train five times a week. If that amount of training is impossible for you, choose the right number from the list and multiply your BMR by that.

Thereafter, gradually build up to training five times a week, as that will ensure you get the best out of the programme.

For those of you doing little exercise, the TDEE figure is going to be quite high, but do not panic. It gives a good starting point to move down from. If, on the other hand, you start low, you have nowhere to go when the time comes to drop calories. Trying to train and survive off 1000 calories, for example, is dangerous and will make you feel terrible. Also, if you train for a period of time at a deficit, at some point you will stop getting results. You will then have to tweak things again, perhaps by dropping 100 calories, which is going from bad to worse.

IF YOUR GOAL IS FAT LOSS

Take your newly found TDEE – 3000 calories, for example. You then start the training programme and drop 100 calories per week until you start seeing your body change. Stop when you are getting to just above your BMR. You want to have a small amount of calories left over for training. Do not try to drop by this total amount all in one go. It's important to do it gradually and monitor how you get on. For some of you it may take four weeks or more to see changes, but stick with it.

Once you have reached minus 500 calories of your TDEE, which in this example would now be 2500 calories, stay at that level for two weeks, then take your measurements. I explain how to do this in chapter two. Continue with the same number of calories for another two weeks, so four weeks in total, then measure again. This would mean that you have dropped 100 calories a week from your original figure until you start to see change, or for a maximum of five weeks. Then spend four weeks at the point you have seen changes. Track your changes by taking your measurements every two weeks. If you stop seeing results or are still struggling to lose weight after dropping your calories by 500 drop another 100 calories – down to 2400 calories per day. Go another two weeks and measure again. If your body still does not change to the point you want, drop another 100 calories and repeat as before making sure that you are monitoring everything you are doing.

Note: Women should not drop more than 800 calories, and men more than 1200, off their total TDEE. Going below those amounts for more than even a few days is not advised, and it's certainly not a good idea in the long- term it causes adverse physiological effects, including disruption of the metabolism and thyroid function. If you have any concerns, don't drop below your BMR on its own. This is the figure that does not include any activity – this is just what it takes to survive.

If, after completing all the steps given here, you still see no gains, your training stimulus is probably wrong. This means you are either not training hard enough, or you are not taking enough rest, or you are letting things such as stress impact your results. A possible solution is to do more cardio work throughout the week – say, two sessions a day – or to use one of your days off for extra cardio.

What will you be eating for fat loss?

There is no need to worry about feeling deprived. For fat loss you will be having four meals a day with an option of one snack.

In simple terms, on the days you train you will eat a meal post workout that is high in protein and carbohydrate. For all the other meals in the day you will be eating high protein, low carbohydrate and moderate to high fats. The recipe section of the book (see page 219) offers a wide variety of options high-carb and low-carb meals, so head to that chapter for inspiration, and to learn that eating healthily can be super-tasty.

If you can't eat or don't feel like eating straight after training, you can have a whey protein shake post workout, or as an extra snack (see page 296). Without contradicting my constant message that wholefoods are better than supplements, taking a supplement can also come in handy when you just can't face a proper meal. See page 208 for further information about supplements and how to use them.

IF YOUR GOAL IS MUSCLE GAIN

To build muscle and gain weight you need to create a calorie surplus. In other words, you need to eat more than your basic requirement so that you have spare calories to fuel your exercise and new tissue building. Not eating enough is the single biggest reason for people failing to get results from the gym, or to see changes from their diet.

Once you have found out your TDEE, let's say 2500 calories, you need to add 250 calories for one week as soon as you start training. Leave it at this level for two weeks, then take your measurements.

For the third week add another 250 calories to your total. This will mean you have added 500 calories to your TDEE over three weeks. Go for another two weeks, then take your measurements again. If you don't see any lean gains, add another 250 calories to your TDEE over the next week (you would then be eating 3250 calories in this example). Stay at that level for two weeks and measure again. Continue this process until you see the gains you want. There is no limit to the number of calories you can add.

All the additional calories must be added gradually. Do not just start eating 500 calories more than you are now on day one: you need to increase things slowly to avoid gaining unwanted weight.

Throughout this time it is really important to monitor your body fat (see page 42). If you start to put on too much, you might need to drop things down by 100 calories, or play with the amounts of protein, carbs and fats you are eating.

If, after completing all the steps given here, you still see no gains, you are probably not training hard enough, or you are not taking enough rest, or you are letting things such as stress impact your results.

What will you be eating for muscle gain?

To build muscle, you will be eating a LOT of food – five meals a day plus one snack. **(The reason meals are split is for ease of consumption. If you can eat your healthy calories in fewer meals then feel free.)**

Every meal you have will contain carbohydrates and high amounts of protein, plus some fats. The recipe chapter (see pages 219) has a selection of meal ideas that fit this bill, and from them you can devise the kind of meals you will enjoy.

As the amount of food you are required to eat is very substantial, you will need to build up your intake gradually. I don't expect you to be eating massive amounts from day one. As ever, do be sure to get most of your calories from proper food. The rule is eat first, supplements later. However, if you are trying to gain muscle for the first time and have never really eaten more than two or three meals a day, it's going to be hard. In this case, some protein shakes (such as those on page 296) can help you to get the extra calories into your body.

A FINAL WORD TO BEGINNERS

Whatever your goal – losing weight or building muscle – please remember to monitor what you are doing from the very beginning. Chapter 2 outlines the best ways to do this (see page 40).

When you have finished the 8-week or 12-week training plan, you might decide to get a bit more serious about nutrition – in which case, I advise you to read the whole of this chapter and learn about macros. These are the component parts of the food you eat, and getting the right balance of them is the next step up in achieving your goal.

MORE ADVANCED NUTRITION

If you are not a beginner to fitness training, or are already knowledgeable about nutrition, the text that follows is aimed at you.

Let's be clear – you can't create a fit body just by training or just by nutrition. The two must work in tandem. As the cliché puts it, you can't out-train a bad diet.

There are so many different ways to put together a nutrition plan that works for you. Just as you need to set goals when beginning the fitness programme, you need to work out exactly what kind of results you want your nutrition plan to achieve. It's easy to find out what works for others – it's all over the internet. The key thing is to find what works for you and stick with it.

Some people say they train and eat well during the week, but let their hair down at weekends, and claim this routine works well for them. In many ways it will, because as long as you do some training and cardiovascular work, you will be helping your health and general body maintenance. However, these people are also the first to say that they never quite get the results they want: they just can't shift that lower abdominal fat or those bingo wings. That's because they are managing rather than developing their body. The fact is that if you do just the minimum with your diet, you will get minimal results, it's as simple as that.

Let me now dispel some other myths and misinformation surrounding fitness. For example, to the best of my knowledge, exercises have not yet been invented that can blast away that tyre of fat around your middle, but you still come across trainers and companies trying to sell you routines or equipment that claim to do just that. The fact

is, you could do abs exercises every day for 20 years and still have that body fat. In simple terms, if you want to see definition of your abdominal muscles, you need to reduce your body fat, and that's achieved through hard training and, more importantly, eating well.

Conversely, if you want to build muscle, you need to feed your body well in both quality and quantity. Undereating merely cheats you out of the results that you could be getting, and is probably the most common problem I come across. This nutrition programme will help to correct that.

Another myth I want to dispel is that eating healthily is expensive. Don't believe it! This idea is often put around by those who just don't understand what constitutes healthy eating. Of course you can spend a fortune on 'bespoke' products, but it is perfectly possible to get everything you need at a fraction of the cost.

I remember watching a TV programme where a woman had convinced herself that she was gluten intolerant. (Of course, some people genuinely are, but it has become something of a fashion to go gluten- or dairy-free. I am intolerant to just one thing, and that is bullshit.) The presenter followed the woman around the supermarket, watching her buy all the expensive health-foods and gluten-free products she considered necessary. Among them was 'gluten-free' white rice, which is nonsense, because white rice has no gluten in it anyway. She paid a ridiculous premium to eat normal rice.

As for other gluten-free products, be aware that a lot of them are higher in fat, salt or sugar than regular products. Also, recent research suggests that cutting gluten out of your diet, unless you really need to, may increase the risk of diabetes and heart disease. My advice, then, is to avoid these special products at all costs, unless you genuinely need them.

Buying simple animal proteins (or meat-free alternatives if you wish), plus carbohydrates and seasonal fruit and vegetables, is not expensive. In fact, these items are cheaper than ready-meals and take little longer to prepare. So be patient and clever with how you shop, and you could save money and eat better.

The following nutrition advice is wide-ranging and suitable for everyone, whether you are looking to lose weight and lean up, or to build muscle. Whatever your goal, here you will find the tools to create your own diet plan that will serve you not just for the 12 weeks of my fitness programme, but for the rest of your life.

Please understand one thing: you can't eat doughnuts and ice cream every day and get in shape. That might sound pretty obvious, but go on Instagram or Google and it's only too easy to find mainstream nutrition 'experts' saying that you can. It might be possible if you are already in killer shape, but for those who aren't, it's important to do things the right way, as outlined in this plan.

Getting your nutrition right is neither especially complicated nor difficult to grasp. The hardest thing is actually putting it in place and keeping to it. There is no escaping the fact that eating well and often is hard work. It requires you to plan ahead and have the right food on hand, or it will be difficult to avoid the temptation of eating 'bad' food.

Dedication to this approach will separate those who get results from those who just play around.

In this chapter I have tried hard to make the eating side of *Perfect Fit* easy to comprehend and straightforward to tailor to your lifestyle and budget. It's not rocket science and shouldn't be treated as such. All I ask is that you read the instructions and commit 100 per cent to getting things right. You might find that you are asked to eat more food than you ever have before, which is counter-intuitive if your goal is to lose weight, but don't be alarmed. It does make sense, and your results will show that.

Remember that getting your nutrition right is a gradual process, requiring time and patience. You can't just eat yourself to an amazing body straight away. It's important that you don't try to eat the volumes of food required right away because you won't be ready for it. You need to make changes gradually, and I will explain how to do that.

If you are doubtful about the importance of diet and think that just training hard will be enough, think again. Diet accounts for 60 per cent of everything you want to achieve from *Perfect Fit*. And remember too that a good diet is essential in general for good health.

I find it's helpful to think of nutrition as like making a deposit in a bank account. Each time you eat well, you put money in; each time you make poor food choices, you take money out. The idea is to build up a healthy bank balance and realise that one bad day of spending won't ruin weeks of hard work. Make too many withdrawals, though, and you will go bankrupt. So invest wisely in yourself and your body. If you do, the results will come.

HOW TO GET STARTED

It is really important to build an understanding of how you normally eat because this provides a starting point from which you can move on. You may never have thought of tracking what you put into your body, but it's essential because memory is fallible. You might recall what you had to eat yesterday or the day before, but you wouldn't be sure of the amounts and exact composition of those meals. The protein, fat and carb content would definitely be hazy. Tracking your food can be an eye-opening process, and explain why you aren't in quite the shape you want.

As I discovered myself, half the food I was at one time consuming wasn't quite as good as I thought. I believed I was eating relatively 'clean', focusing on single-ingredient foods and avoiding 'junk', such as chocolate and cakes. I was shocked to learn that my fat levels were way higher than I imagined. I really needed to tighten things up. Here's how I went about it.

TRACKING YOUR FOOD

The easiest way to get to grips with what you eat is to track your food by keeping a diary or using an app such as MyFitnessPal. You simply make a note of what you eat at every meal, including the amounts. The advantage of the app is that it will immediately give you a breakdown of the calorie, protein, carbohydrate and fat content of each food.

The other great feature of MyFitnessPal is a barcode scanner, which allows you to check what food contains before you buy it. Do this for a week and you will get a clear picture of what you are eating and the calories you are consuming.

If you don't have a smartphone, you can download an online food diary template to your computer. It will be a lot more time-consuming to fill in, but at the end of five days you will get a picture of what's going in your body.

Whichever method you choose to track your food, make sure you are super-honest. You don't have to share the data with anyone but yourself, so there is no point in cheating – you'll simply spoil your results. Look at it this way: if it makes terrible reading, that's good because you can easily improve it.

TIPS FOR STARTING TO CHANGE YOUR DIET

Earlier in this book, I made it clear that you don't need to buy loads of special equipment or attend an upmarket gym in order to get results. The same frugal approach applies to nutrition. You will need to start eating well from the very beginning, but that doesn't mean going mad and changing everything at once. It is a gradual process, and changing your diet is something you will need to feel your way into. It will take a bit of time to go from apprentice to nutrition Jedi.

Make a couple of small, simple changes and stick with them

For example, during the first week or so, you could start eating breakfast, something that many people skip. If you don't already eat a protein-based breakfast within 30 minutes of waking up, you should definitely add it to your daily meal plan. This initial injection of protein (eggs, red meat or oily fish) can make a massive difference to your health, as it goes to your immune system rather than your muscles. Who doesn't want a stronger immune system?

If you start the day well you will be able to concentrate and work better throughout the day.

Divide your diet into pre-training and post-training meals

This would mean eating four to five times a day, but one of those meals would be a snack.

If you are looking for fat loss, a calorie deficit is your primary concern, as far as macros go, carbohydrates should be in your post training meals ONLY, the rest of the time fats should replace carbs in your meals.

For muscle building, you should be having protein, carbs and fats throughout the day with all your meals. The reason we split meals up is so you can eat all the calories needed without feeling bloated, unable to train and more importantly allowing your body to digest things properly. Your body can only digest a maximum amount of macros over time. There is still a lot of research going into what these amounts are.

Boost your intake of all vegetables

This certainly holds true during the first couple of weeks, no matter what your goal, and is actually worth doing for the rest of the plan too. It's always good to look into your supermarket trolley or down at your plate and see a wide variety of colours, as this is the best way of ensuring you get a good range of vitamins and minerals. Vegetables are a great source of micronutrients, such as vitamin C, iron, potassium and folate, while their phytochemicals, such as lycopene and beta-carotene, offer real benefits to long-term health and help to reduce the risk of many diseases associated with ageing. Vegetables are also good sources of fibre, which is essential for maintaining gut health and preventing constipation and other digestive problems.

Have a good source of protein with every meal

There are loads of choices available, but chicken, red meat, fish, dairy and eggs are the best as they contain no additives or anything that nature didn't intend.

For your carb options, opt for single-ingredient foods, such as potatoes, rice, squashes and yams. This keeps things simple when you are starting out on your healthy-eating journey, and lets you know exactly what you are putting into your body. Potatoes, for example, are exactly as nature intended: they contain no additives or preservatives. You can also include pulses (beans, peas and lentils), and grains such as quinoa and barley. These are all natural, and add variety, flavour and important nutrients to your diet.

FOODS TO AVOID

The following list might seem obvious, but a reminder can be helpful. Here's a list of what you should avoid:

>> **Processed food** – junk food, fast food, ready-meals, cakes, pastries, biscuits and sweets.
>> **Refined foods** – white pasta, white bread, white sugar, etc. I don't mind if you eat a lot of white rice, as we aren't trying to prepare you for a photoshoot, and it's a great and easy carb to have. If you are also trying to build muscle, you can be a little more relaxed about eating refined products.
>> **Sugar-sweetened fizzy drinks** – the sugar content is always incredibly high, and has no nutritional content, so avoid sugary drinks at all costs.

Do not skip meals or allow yourself to get over-hungry. This will adversely affect your results, as you won't be adequately fuelling your training or recovery. It also means you will be more likely to fall off the wagon and reach for 'bad' food, or eat too quickly and thus overeat. Your body isn't stupid, so if you don't feed it well, it will start to crave what it's missing. If your blood sugar is low, your energy level will be low too, and you will start wanting sweet fatty foods, such as chocolate.

Failing to eat, or eating badly, can also have a massive impact on behaviour and mood. For example, children who eat loads of sugary cereal before school, or skip breakfast altogether, often misbehave or can't concentrate. Adults too can be moody and lethargic.

An alarming fact is that if you don't fuel your body, it will start to eat itself, drawing on its stores of fat and muscle. This is far from desirable, so my message is, don't go hungry and always make sure you eat.

FAT BOMBING

To some people, the term 'fat bombing' refers to a ketogenic diet, which is high in fat and low in carbs. That is not what I'm talking about here. The sense in which I'm using it refers to clearing your kitchen of unhealthy fatty foods by giving them away.

At the start of any programme designed to change your life, it's all too easy to get carried away with the thought of a new you. You rush out and buy all the healthy foods, only to succumb to eating those unhealthy foods still lingering in your cupboards when things get difficult.

We all know that temptation is incredibly difficult to resist, so before you go shopping for new stuff, get rid of the old. Clear your kitchen cupboards of all those treats intended for either you or the kids and give them away – to friends, family, food banks ... you choose. Simply 'bomb' them with fat. Once temptation has been removed from your cupboards, all you will have to hand in times of weakness (which happen to everyone) is good food.

GETTING TO GRIPS WITH NUTRITION

As you read on, you will find the nutrition information becomes a little more complicated, perhaps even a bit daunting. You can refer back to the simple fat loss and nutrition guide for beginers earlier in the book. Please trust me that it is actually very simple – it just takes some concentration at first. However, if you struggle with some of the suggestions, you can simply follow the main principles of the nutrition plan and build up to the more complex stuff as you become more confident.

To understand what constitutes good food, you need to know a few technical terms, so here are the principal ones.

MACRONUTRIENTS

Known as 'macros' for short, macronutrients are the compounds we need to eat in relatively large amounts to provide us with energy. These are split into three different food groups: protein, carbohydrate and fat.

Protein (e.g. meat, poultry, fish, eggs, dairy, beans with grains, pulses, tofu and nuts with grains)
Protein forms the building blocks for cells

in the body. It is needed for repairing and building body tissues and structures. 1g of protein contains 4 calories.

This plan at times recommends a high protein intake because training involves damaging and breaking down muscle tissue. This in turn sets off a process known as protein synthesis, whereby the body creates new muscle proteins to replace and add to the damaged tissues.

In fact, proteins contribute towards the growth and repair of many areas of the body, not just muscles. They play an important role in making amino acids, which are essential in the production of hormones.

It must be noted that doing exercise, particularly resistance training, increases the protein needs of the body. Your best options to fulfil this increased requirement are animal-based proteins, such as meat, fish, eggs and dairy, but plant-based proteins, such as quinoa, beans and nuts (perhaps in the form of nut butters), also make a useful contribution. Note that beans and nuts are not complete proteins and need to be mixed with grains to make them complete.

Carbohydrate (e.g. oats, potatoes, rice, pasta, wholegrains)

This is the chief source of energy for all body functions and muscular exertion. 1g of carbohydrate contain 4 calories.

Wholegrain, unrefined carbohydrates contain fibre, which is important for bowel function and the body's absorption of glucose. Gut health is often overlooked, but is essential for getting the best results from your diet.

Carbohydrates are the preferred fuel source of the muscles. During high-intensity exercise, the muscles use glucose to drive muscular contractions and replenish glycogen stores (glycogen is the storage form of glucose).

More carbohydrates are required on training days and in meals directly post-workout. You should aim to reach your carb requirements through wholegrains, oats, brown rice, sweet potatoes and pulses, even some wholemeal bread, while avoiding highly processed sources, such as biscuits and sweets. If you are trying to build just muscle, you can be a little more relaxed over your sources of carbohydrates.

Fat (e.g. nuts, eggs, avocado, seeds, coconut oil, fatty fish)

The human body cannot function without fat. It maintains healthy cell membranes, while facilitating the absorption of fat-soluble vitamins (A, D, E, K) and the production of hormones. 1g of fat contains roughly 9 calories.

Dietary fat is an essential part of any diet because it provides essential fatty acids, such as omega-3, that cannot be synthesised in the body. It also provides the highest calories-per-gram contribution of energy out of the three macronutrients. Fat is essential for sustaining longer, slower and lower-intensity exercise, such when you are working, walking around or even sleeping.

MICRONUTRIENTS

There are two broad categories of micronutrient: vitamins and minerals. Although they have very little, if any, calorific value, and are needed in only tiny amounts, they are essential for healthy growth and metabolism, as well as immune support and brain function.

FATS GOOD AND BAD

It's important to distinguish between the different types of fat, as there are some you need to avoid or least cut back on:

» **Essential fatty acids (EFAs)** are types of polyunsaturated fat that help to lower blood cholesterol and prevent blood clots, reduce inflammaton and help with recovery. Omega-3 is found in linseed, soya and walnut oils, while omega-6 is found in corn, safflower, soya and sunflower oils. Both are also found in oily fish, such as herring, mackerel and salmon. If, for one reason or another, you can't eat fish, you could take an omega-3 supplement that is derived from algae.

As many people tend to use vegetable margarines and to cook with vegetable oil, they ingest much higher levels of omega-6 than omega-3, and this imbalance is not ideal. If possible, try to keep your intake of both around the same.

» **Monounsaturated fats** include olive oil, rapeseed oil, nuts, seeds and avocados, and are considered healthier than saturates because they reduce levels of harmful cholesterol in the blood.

» **Polyunsaturated fats** are found in plant foods, such as sunflower oil, and fish such as salmon and mackerel. They are considered beneficial because they lower levels of cholesterol in the blood to an even greater degree than monounsaturates.

» **Saturated fats** tend to be found in animal products, such as meat, butter and lard, and have long had a reputation for doing us harm by furring up the arteries with cholesterol, which can lead to heart attacks and other health problems. Their poor reputation has now been at least partially revised because it turns out that saturated fats – in moderation – play a vital role in hormone production and may help to destroy viruses.

» **Trans fats** start life as unsaturated fats, but they behave like saturates when processed with hydrogen, which is done to increase their stability and shelf life. They are easy to avoid because they are generally found in processed foods, such as cakes, biscuits and ready-meals. These days many food manufacturers are committed to phasing out the use of trans fats.

HOW TO CALCULATE YOUR MACROS

We are all different, so our individual macro needs are different too. The major factors affecting your daily macros (the amount of protein, fat and carbohydrates you need per day) are your body weight and your body type. As discussed on page 20, your inherited genes play a role in not getting the body you want, or for finding it harder to achieve your goals. Losing weight or gaining it is simply harder for some than for others. Once you understand your body type, you can look out for these things and either add or take away from your plan. In general, the heavier you are, the more calories or macro intake you require.

In order to calculate your macros, you need to work out your BMR and TDEE, as explained on page 185.

The next step I strongly recommend is to download MyFitnessPal to your smartphone. This app allows you to input the food you're eating, notes how many calories it contains, gives a breakdown of its macro content, and from all this information it shows your calorie intake for the day and what proportion of each macro those calories contain. If you have never worked out your BMR/TDEE or have no idea what amounts you eat in a day, MyFitnessPal makes it really easy to find out. Once you have decided on your goal and followed my steps, you will then add this information to the app, and aim to hit all the targets every day. You will be able to see what the foods you are eating contain in terms of protein, carbs and fat

HOW TO WORK OUT MACRO SPLITS FOR FAT LOSS

Now you have an idea of the calories you should be eating, you need to work out the percentage of macronutrients they need to contain. This will help you to construct your eating plan.

First a little background on how this calculation works. Per gram, protein and carbohydrate both contribute 4 kcal of energy, whereas fat contributes 9 kcal. To work out the protein, carb and fat requirements of each phase of training, please use the following guidelines:

1 Multiply your daily calories by the percentage of each macro (if 40 per cent is required, multiply the total calories by 0.4).
2 Divide by the number of calories the macro source contributes (for protein and carb divide by 4, for fat divide by 9).
3 The resulting figure is the macro requirement in grams.

When aiming for fat loss, macro requirements vary, depending on whether you are resting or training.

On training days you are eating only carbs post-training. For all the other meals on training days you are having high protein and moderate fats. This means that you will end up having all your starchy carbs at one meal. The remaining meals will consist of green vegetables and other incidentals.

For example, protein powder contains some carbs, as does fat free Greek yoghurt etc, however these are not to be fretted over.

Rest days are slightly different in relation to carbs. Instead of starchy carbs, such as potatoes and rice, you will get your carbs from non-starchy sources, such as some vegetables, yoghurt, dark chocolate, berries and peanut butter.

Here is an example of fat loss macro splits for someone with a daily calorie requirement of 2000:

Training day macro splits
» Protein 40%
» Carbohydrates (starchy, i.e. high-carb foods) 30%
» Fats 30%

Rest day macro splits
» Protein 40%
» Carbohydrates (non-starchy, i.e. low-carb foods) 30%
» Fats 30%

The gram amounts you require are calculated as follows, the emboldened figure being our notional 2000 kcal requirement, which you will replace with your own:

Protein
0.4 x **2000** = 800
800 ÷ 4 = 200
So 200g of protein is required on training days.

Carbohydrate
0.3 x **2000** = 600
600 ÷ 4 = 150

So 150g of carbohydrate is required on training days.

Fat
0.3 x **2000** = 600
600 ÷ 9 = 66
So 66g of fat is required on training days.

Just remember that 150g of carbs, for example, does not mean simply 150g of potatoes. That amount will supply only 25g of carbs, so you would be way short for the day.

This is where an app comes in useful to work out how much of a particular food is needed to give you your specific macro requirement. With our trusty friend MyFitnessPal, you enter your calories and your macro splits, fill in the foods, and it tells you how much you have to eat and what the protein, carb and fat content is.

Why do I keep banging on about hitting your macros and calories? Simply because it's important to ensure your body is getting the correct amount of energy and macronutrients at the correct times. If you don't get this right, it can really slow your progress with fat loss, but, even worse, it can push you into a catabolic state, where your body starts breaking down its own muscles. Muscles are hard enough to build as it is, so you don't want to have them eaten up. You need to fuel your body properly and burn the unwanted fat while retaining the muscle.

HOW MANY MEALS SHOULD I EAT FOR FAT LOSS?

You will be eating four meals a day, one of them can be a snack if you have limited calories left. We have some snack options for you to follow, but if you are really pushed for time, a simple protein shake will do. There is a section on supplements that will give you some recommendations (see page 213). On the days that you are training you will be eating a meal with carbs post-training. The rest of your meals will consist of fats, vegetables and protein.

PLATE COMPOSITION FOR FAT LOSS

What sort of thing should you see on your plate? Try to imagine it like a pie chart. On training days you are having carbs post-workout, so the biggest slice of the pie will be protein, the next biggest will be carbohydrates, and the smallest slices will be fats and vegetables.

For every other meal on training days and non-training days the biggest slice is again protein, the second biggest slices are fats and vegetables, and the smallest will be carbs (non-starchy ones, such as green veg and other incidentals).

Two sample eating plans are given on page 205 – one for a day when training in the morning, and another for a day when you train in the evening. However, before you look at these, please read the following text about fasting.

TRAINING FASTED

This is simply training on an empty stomach, which some in the fitness world believe is the best way to burn fat. You would do it just after waking up, without having put any food into your body. Note that it should be done only with cardio or HIIT, never for lifting weights.

The thinking behind this approach is that your body has been given no fuel, so it will use its fat stores to get through the training session. This is not scientifically proven, but a lot of people swear by it.

I have trained fasted a few times when I wanted to maximise my fat burning, but it's not something that I do normally. You are welcome to give it a try and see how you get on.

The best way to train fasted is to hydrate with water, then, if you can stomach it (some can't), take a pre-trainer supplement or you could try using BCAAs (Branch Chain Amino Acid). The idea behind them is to stop catabolism, where your body breaks down muscle (see page 273). You will need the energy boost it gives to get through training.

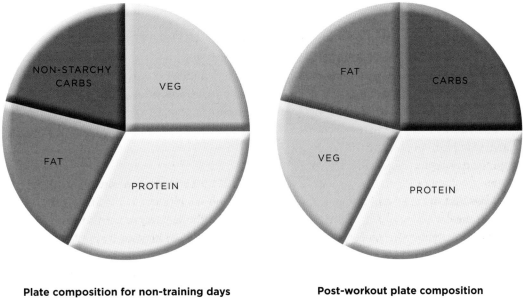

Plate composition for non-training days

Post-workout plate composition for training days

SAMPLE MEAL PLANS

The plans shown on these pages are very loose, intended only to give you an idea of what your day should look like. Do not try to follow them. Your macros and calories will be very different, so you need to construct your own plan, which might include some of the recipes mentioned, but also some modified versions. (See the recipe chapter on page 219 for ideas that you can tailor to your needs.)

Sample meal plan when
training before breakfast
>> *Morning* – no foods
>> *Training session* – fasted (optional)
>> *Pre-workout* – water and optional pre-workout supplement or coffee
>> *During workout* – optional BCAA drinks or water

>> *Post-workout* – protein shake, consisting of whey protein and some carbs
Meal 1 – high-carb breakfast, e.g. eggs, toast, oats (I would eat the oats as porridge made with water, but milk can be used if you prefer, just make sure you include the milk in your macros.)
Meal 2 – low-carb lunch, e.g. lean mince chilli cooked with coconut oil or whatever oil you choose
Meal 3 – low-carb dish, e.g. Asian mango salad with roast chicken (see page 254)
Meal 4 – low-carb dinner, e.g. Fillet of beef with spinach yoghurt sauce and rocket salad (see page 274)

Sample meal plan when training post-breakfast

Meal 1 – low-carb breakfast, e.g. Steak with eggs and watercress sauce (see page 230)
Training session: pre-workout – water and optional pre-workout supplement, shake or coffee
» *During workout* – optional BCAA drinks with water
» *Post-workout* – protein shake with carbs, e.g. whey protein
Meal 2 – high-carb lunch, e.g. Grilled chicken with edamame bean and cashew salad (see page 238)
Meal 3 – low-carb snack, e.g. Peanut butter energy balls (see page 294)
Meal 4 – low-carb dinner, e.g. Roasted salmon with peas and asparagus, (see page 275)

Sample meal plan when training in the evening

Meal 1 – low-carb breakfast, e.g. Turkey escalope with spinach chimichurri (see page 231)
Meal 2 – low-carb lunch, e.g. Smoked mackerel salad (see page 251)
Meal 3 – low-carb snack, e.g. Spinach and feta hummus with crudités (see page 294)
» *Training session: pre-workout* – water and optional pre-workout supplement, shake or coffee
» *During workout* – optional BCAA drinks or water
» *Post-workout* – protein shake with carbs, e.g. whey protein
Meal 4 – high-carb dinner, e.g. Turkey katsu curry with brown rice (see page 260)

Sample meal plan for a non-training day

Meal 1 – low-carb breakfast, e.g. Roasted tomatoes, scrambled eggs and Parmesan (see page 231)
Meal 2 – low-carb lunch, e.g. Crispy Vietnamese beef with peanut salad (see page 250)
Meal 3 – low-carb snack, e.g. Chocolate brownie (see page 295)
Meal 4 – low-carb dinner, e.g. Lamb in yoghurt with carrot salad (see page 280)
Optional – low-carb protein shake (just whey)

All the recipe ideas above come from Chapter 7 (page 219), so head over there to get even more great ideas for creating deliciousness in the kitchen.

HOW TO WORK OUT MACRO SPLITS FOR MUSCLE GAIN

To gain muscle you will need to put your body into a calorie surplus to enable you to grow. As before, start by multiplying your BMR by 1.55 (because you are training five times a day) to get your TDEE. Take this figure and in week 1, multiply the figure above by 1.1 (10% surplus). In weeks 2–12, you will need to multiply the above figure by 1.2 (20% surplus).

If you have worked things out correctly, you will know that you have two different calorie targets – one for the initial week and another for the remaining weeks of the programme.

Unlike fat loss, where you have different macro splits for training days and rest days, muscle gain requires you to eat consistently all the time.

The ideal splits are:
» Protein 40%
» Carbohydrate 40%
» Fats 20%

In this case, the gram amounts are calculated as follows, the notional requirement of 3000 kcl being in bold.

Protein
0.4 x **3000** = 1200
1200 ÷ **4** = 300

So 300g of protein is required on both training and rest days.

Carbohydrate
0.4 x **3000** = 1200
1200 ÷ **4** = 300

So 300g of carbohydrate is required on both training and rest days.

Fat
0.2 x **3000** = 600
600 ÷ **9** = 67
So 67g of fat is required on both training and rest days.

Just remember that 200g of protein, for example, does not mean simply 200g of chicken. That will supply only 40g of protein, so you would be way short. As usual, MyFitnessPal app comes in useful for calculating things accurately.

HOW MANY MEALS SHOULD I EAT FOR MUSCLE GAIN?

I suggest having four meals a day in the first week plus a protein shake. This new nutrition plan will take some time to get used to, and if you haven't been eating properly or enough, you will find it quite hard.

As the calories increase, I suggest going up to five meals plus a protein shake with carbs. You should find that all the activity you are doing has increased your appetite. The protein shake is not mandatory and can be replaced by food, but once you are eating and training as you should be, it will sometimes be hard to consume all the food you need. Consult the information about supplements (see page 214), which covers what you should take and why.

Week 1 (intro phase as per training guide)
4 meals per day + high-carb shake
(see Chapter 7 for recipe ideas)

Weeks 2–12 (as per training guide)
4 or 5 meals per day + high-carb shake
(you might end up having two shakes a day if you train early in the morning; see Chapter 7 for recipe ideas)

This is going to be an extremely intense phase of the training plan, so it's important to have the correct fuel to perform at your best for each and every workout. Here you will increase your meals to five a day, as well as having a high-carb protein shake. During this phase you will be on a 20 per cent calorie surplus.

Carbohydrate is the preferred substrate to fuel the muscles, so to optimise results, to provide the energy required to fuel a heavy workout, and to replace glycogen stores post-workout, **you will be using a macro split of 40/40/20 on your training days**. I am suggesting five meals a day because of the volume of food that you are being required to eat. If you can eat your daily calories in fewer healthy meals, please feel free.

PLATE COMPOSITION FOR MUSCLE GAIN

Most of your meals should consist of a protein source, say two chicken breasts. Beside that you need a similar-sized portion of carbohydrates, such as rice or potatoes, or whatever carb source you have selected. The smallest portion will be vegetables (non-starchy carbs) and fats (such as nuts, oils, olives). The amounts of each item will be based on your macros, which you will have worked out from the formula on page 207.

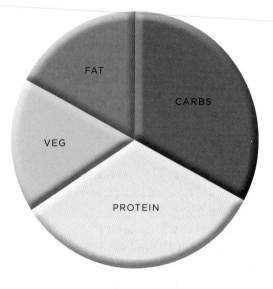

Plate composition for muscle gain

SAMPLE EATING PLANS FOR MUSCLE BUILDING

Sample eating plan for
training before breakfast

>> *Morning* – hydration; protein shake with carbs; optional pre-workout

>> *Training session:* water and optional BCAAs during workout

>> *Post-workout* – protein shake with carbs (or you can eat a meal straight away if you can stomach it)

Meal 1 – high-carb breakfast, e.g. Ham, feta and fig flatbread (see page 222)

Meal 2 – high-carb lunch, e.g. Turkey koftas with Persian rice (see page 240)

Meal 3 – high-carb snack, e.g. Coffee and chocolate bites (see page 290)

Meal 4 – high-carb meal, e.g. Spaghetti and pancetta, chilli, parsley and Parmesan (see page 267)

Meal 5 – high-carb dinner, e.g. Chicken, coconut, chickpea and spinach curry with pilau rice (see page 269)

Sample eating plan for
training post-breakfast

Meal 1 – high-carb breakfast, e.g. Corn and chilli fritters (see page 224)

>> *Training session:* pre-workout – hydration; optional pre-trainer

>> *During workout* – water and optional BCAAs

>> *Post-workout* – protein shake with carbs (or you can eat a meal straight away if you can stomach it)

Meal 2 – high-carb lunch, e.g. Chilli and lime chicken with Thai noodle salad (see page 242)

Meal 3 – high-carb snack, e.g. Chickpea and chocolate cookie (see page 288)

Meal 4 – high-carb meal, e.g. Halloumi with mixed beans and pomegranate (see page 239)

Meal 5 – high-carb dinner, e.g. Fillet of cod with roasted squash polenta (see page 268)

Sample eating plan for
training in the evening

Meal 1 – high-carb breakfast, e.g. Coconut porridge (see page 227)

Meal 2 – high-carb lunch, e.g. Chicken, chorizo, butterbean and sweet potato salad (see page 247)

Meal 3 – high-carb snack, e.g. Roasted salt and chilli almonds (see page 288)

Meal 4 – high-carb meal, e.g. Harissa-grilled sardines with walnut potato salad (see page 265)

>> *Training session:* pre-workout – hydration; optional pre-trainer

>> *During workout* – water and optional BCAAs

>> *Post-workout* – protein shake with carbs (or you can eat a meal straight away if you can stomach it)

Meal 5 – high-carb dinner, e.g. Mini chicken pastilla (see page 270)

As you can see, whether you are eating to lose or gain weight, it requires a lot of thought and time. It's one thing to know what to eat, it's another thing to actually get it all sorted and cook the food. Overleaf are some tips to help you.

TIPS FOR GETTING YOUR FOOD ON TRACK

>> **Prepare your food in advance.** This will make life much easier, as well as ensuring you stay on track. Aim to prepare for the day ahead either the night before or at breakfast time.

>> **Buy lots of plastic food boxes.** Filled with the delicious food you've prepared in advance, these will be your new best friends for the next 12 weeks. Just tuck a few into a coolbag when you set off for the day so that you always have good food at hand. It will mean you're not reaching for unhealthy sandwich options or junk food.

>> **Have a big cook-up on Sundays.** You can then freeze the meals in plastic containers and bring them out when needed.

>> **Multiply the amounts you cook.** For example, if you need one chicken breast for dinner, it's just as easy to cook three more for the following day. And while you're about it, cook extra veg, rice or whatever else you're having with it.

>> **Learn to eat out healthily.** If you have the MyFitnessPal app on your phone, you can check out what's on offer in a restaurant and get a rough idea of the protein, carb and fats in each dish. I always go for fish when I have to eat out and I am on my nutrition plan. Unless it comes in batter with a side of chips, fish is a pretty safe bet.

>> **Buy tailor-made meals.** This is an expensive option, but useful if you really don't have time to shop or cook for yourself. There are plenty of food delivery services that will create meals to your exact macro requirements. Some simply provide the measured ingredients for you to cook as you wish. Others supply ready-cooked meals that you just heat up. I have used many of these companies and found them really good, but the food can become repetitive and boring. Also, if you don't cook for yourself, you won't ever learn how.

>> **Discover the joys of online food shopping.** If you hate going to the shops or feel you simply don't have time to go out and stock up, get into online shopping. Everything can be delivered to your door, so you need never run out of food. It also means there's no excuse to fall off your diet or miss out on making those fitness gains. Just put together a repeat order of chicken, fish, potatoes, veg and rice so you always have the basics to hand.

HEALTHY FOOD SOURCES

It's really important to get some idea of what should be going into your shopping basket in order to build a healthy diet. The following tables, all from verified sources, offer some examples, but once again I suggest you use the app MyFitnessPal to scan packet ingredients and work out what's suitable. It really is the best app on the market, and I assure you that I have no links or vested interest in recommending it.

Protein sources

Per 100g or 100ml, raw	Protein	Carbohydrate	Fat
Almond milk, unsweetened	0.4g	0g	1.1g
Almonds, unsalted	25.4g	6.6g	55.8g
Beef mince (5% fat)	21.0g	0g	6.1g
Beef steak, fillet	21.2g	0g	9.0g
Casein (Maximuscle brand), 1 scoop	24.0g	3.1g	0.8g
Chicken breast, skinless	24.0g	0g	1.1g
Cottage cheese (full-fat)	9.2g	3.0g	6.0g
Egg (1 medium, whole)	7.7g	0.4g	5.5g
Egg white (1 medium)	3.5g	0g	0g
Lamb, lean	20.2g	0g	8.0g
Milk, semi-skimmed	3.4g	4.5g	1.7g
Milk, skimmed	3.4g	4.6g	0.3g
Milk, whole	3.3g	5.4g	3.3g
Peanuts, unsalted	29.6g	11.9g	46.0g
Salmon	20.4g	0g	15.0g
Tuna, fresh	25.2g	0g	1.1g
Turkey breast	24.4g	0g	0.8g
Whey protein, ON brand (30g)	26.7g	3.3g	1.1g
Yoghurt, Greek (0% fat)	10.3g	3.8g	0g
Yoghurt, Greek (full-fat)	5.6g	4.6g	10.2g
Yoghurt, plain (low-fat)	4.7g	7.4g	1.0g

Starchy carbohydrate sources (i.e. high-carb foods)

Per 100g, raw	Protein	Carbohydrate	Fat
Bread, wholemeal	10.3g	40g	2.5g
Brown basmati rice	8g	70g	3g
Butternut squash	1.4g	16.4g	0g
Carrots	1.2g	12.3g	0.3g
Green beans	1g	4g	0g
Pasta, dried	12.4g	72.0g	1.6g
Pilau rice	3.8g	30.7g	3.1g
Porridge oats	5g	27g	3g
Potato, baking	1.0g	18.7g	0g
Potatoes, new	1.5g	10.5g	0.1g
Quinoa	13.1g	68.9	13.1g
Rice cake (7.5g)	0.6g	6.1g	0g
Sweet potato	1.6g	21g	0.1g
White rice, long-grain	7.0g	81g	1.0g

Non-starchy carbohydrate sources (i.e. low-carb foods)

Per 100g, raw	Protein	Carbohydrate	Fat
Asparagus	2.9g	1.9g	0.6g
Berries, mixed	0.9g	5.9g	0.3g
Broccoli	4.3g	3.0g	0.6g
Cabbage	1.1g	5.2g	0.1g
Mushrooms, white	2.5g	0.3g	0.2g
Onions	1.0g	7.6g	0.1g
Tomato (1 small)	0.5g	2.9g	0.1g

Healthy fat sources

Per 100g raw, or as indicated	Protein	Carbohydrate	Fat
Almond butter (15g/1 tbsp)	3.8g	0.9g	8.4g
Avocado (1 medium – 150g)	2.8g	2.7g	29.2g
Coconut oil (15ml/1 tbsp)	0g	0g	11.0g
Mackerel fillet	18.0g	0g	17.9g
Olive oil (15ml/1 tbsp)	0g	0g	11.0g
Peanut butter (15g/1 tbsp)	3.9g	1.9g	7.8g

SUPPLEMENTS

Lots of people ask, 'Are supplements necessary? Will they really help me get results?' As far as I'm concerned, supplements play a role, but a very small one, in training. They are an afterthought, not a priority. At times they can be the icing on the cake, but the cake itself should be just good food. I recommend getting 95 per cent of what you need from balanced, whole foods.

Supplements are not meal replacements; neither are they miracle agents that will suddenly get you into amazing shape. If they do, they are probably illegal and very bad for you. I think they're best viewed as a finishing touch, not a complete means to an end.

The daily diet plan in this book does occasionally suggest using supplements, but not at the expense of good food. Within *Perfect Fit*, I want you to reach a calorific surplus in your diet if you are building muscle, but sometimes it is just not possible to consume as much food as you need. As a consequence, some of the surplus required can come from protein shakes.

Occasionally, supplements can help even if you are looking to lose weight. For example, after a gruelling training session the last thing you want is to force down mounds of food. I have tried it many times but got only halfway through or wished the food would simply disappear. It would have been easier to have a really nutritious shake and I could have eaten well later on.

Of course, eating food, and the initial chewing of it, should take priority over drinking it, not least because your body needs solid food for the digestion to work on. The process extracts enzymes from it, many of which combine to perform key functions in the body. That can only happen if you eat a balanced meal. A whey protein shake, by contrast, contains only a simple protein.

Most of the supplements I take are used just to top things up, or to help me work on deficient areas. I can do this because I have undergone rigorous blood tests to find out the exact areas where I might be deficient. However, even these tests can change, so what can be measured and defined is constantly disputed. Nonetheless, I know what to take to get my required nutrition quickly when I don't have food to hand.

However, this is an area that I am constantly looking to improve and try new things to maximise results and performance.

In addition, I am extremely careful about the supplements I do take. I am constantly being drug-tested, so anything I put into my body needs to be batch tested first.

The supplement world is a bit like the Wild West: so much of it is unregulated and untested. Manufacturers are not obliged to list every single ingredient on the packaging, some cowboy ones don't, and consumers therefore have no real idea of what they are taking. The only way to be sure that supplements are any good is if they have gone through the Informed Sport testing programme. This means the factories themselves are inspected and that everything they produce is batch tested.

Unfortunately, not everything that is tested is of the best quality. It might have impressive packaging, but the ingredients are not top notch. That's one of the reasons that I started my own supplement range. I want to be confident about what I'm putting into my body, and potentially into yours. The bottom line is that you get what you actually pay for as opposed to something rogue that has slipped through the net.

APPROVED SUPPLEMENTS

Following is a list of supplements you might like to consider adding gradually to your nutrition plan and training protocol, but only once you have got on top of your diet by conventional means. Those listed will help with performance, recovery and general health, as well as helping you to reach your macro levels. Among them are some designed to boost your immune system, which can take a hammering when you embark on an intense training programme. There are also some that help to improve sleep, which is very important in helping your recovery from the rigours of training.

Note that I haven't listed any brand names because, based on what I've told you, I want you to do your own research and choose for yourselves. I don't want to be accused of any favouritism.

BCAAs

There are 20 basic amino acids, which are the building blocks of new proteins. However, just three of these are key to initiating protein synthesis. These are leucine, isoleucine and valine, otherwise known as Branch Chain Amino Acids. Some argue that BCAAs are not completely necessary when on a high-calorie diet, but if you have the money, I recommend taking a BCAA product both pre- and during your workout to decrease the chance of your body going into a catabolic state (where it consumes its own muscles) and to promote protein synthesis.

Dosage: As directed by the manufacturer, generally 5–10g pre- and during workout.

Creatine

Far too many schoolboys think creatine has steroid-like qualities that can help to build huge muscles. That is utter rubbish and should be ignored. Creatine occurs naturally in the muscles, but can be supplemented to considerable effect, as it greatly increases the ability to perform explosive work. Many people begin by taking a high dose for a week or so, a period known as a 'loading phase'. During this time the muscles will become saturated with phosphocreatine, the form in which it is stored in muscle cells. The loading phase is then followed by a maintenance phase, a period of taking a lower dose, which is designed to maintain high phosphocreatine levels in the muscles. I suggest, however, that you take a low, unchanging dose over time and you will get to the saturation level without having to ingest a lot at any particular point.

Dosage: As directed by the manufacturer or your nutritionist.

Multivitamins

I have always taken a multivitamin, mainly to support my immune system and to fill any gaps that my diet doesn't cover. There is a lot of talk about whether multivitamins actually work, but for me they do.

Dosage: 1 a day or as directed.

Omega-3 fish oils

Omega-3s – ALA, DHA and EPA – are fatty acids that come from fish and are known to have beneficial effects on the body. They are really good for cognitive function, cardiovascular function and the joints. Supplements containing omega-3s have historically focused on providing a balanced level of these fatty acids, but increasingly experts in sports nutrition are suggesting that higher levels of EPA might be better for sports professionals and highly active individuals who are looking to aid recovery. If you are eating a lot oily fish as part of your diet, you might not need to supplement with fish oils. Those allergic to fish could take an alternative source of omega-3 derived from algae.

Dosage: As directed by the manufacturer or your nutritionist.

Probiotics and Prebiotics

Probiotics are friendly bacteria found in foodstuffs such as yoghurt and kefir, while prebiotics are substances that stimulate the production of beneficial micro-organisms in the gut. A healthy digestive system is really important because it affects how nutrients from food are absorbed, and this in turn can affect the efficiency of the immune system and the removal of waste products. Poor gut health can be a particular issue for older people who haven't eaten well for some time. You will already know if your gut health is less than it should be, so it could be worth trying a high-end probiotic to help repair it.

Dosage: As directed by the manufacturer or your nutritionist.

Vitamin D

A fat-soluble vitamin (technically a prohormone), vitamin D is known for its effects on bone and calcium metabolism. It also plays a role in maintaining the immune system. We get most of our vitamin D from sunlight, which in countries like the UK is quite limited, so many people suffer from a deficiency. This is easy to test for and can be remedied by taking a supplement. One research review noted that boosting vitamin D appeared to bring benefits to physical activity, but the results were not conclusive, and there is still lots of research going on.

Dosage: Opinion varies but Public Health England (PHE) says that adults and children over the age of one year should have 10 micrograms (mcg) of vitamin D every day.

Whey protein

Whey is derived from milk, and its protein content is extracted and dried for use as a supplement. Its great benefits when training are that it is very quick to digest, it initiates protein synthesis (muscle growth) and it's great as a snack. However, if you are lactose intolerant, stick to whey isolates to avoid lactose. Note too that many whey products include poor-quality ingredients or fillers, so always go for the highest-quality brand, ideally Informed Sport tested.

Dosage: Take post-training sessions, when you can't eat a meal within the hour, or if you don't have a good food source to hand.

ZMA

This supplement is a combination of zinc, magnesium and vitamin B6 and is a great recovery aid. Zinc is important for almost all metabolic processes, especially protein synthesis, and helps maintain a healthy immune system. Magnesium helps regulate electrolyte balance, energy production and neuromuscular function. Vitamin B6 helps the nervous system and supports adrenal function, which in turn controls metabolism. ZMA is known to increase the body's production of growth compounds, and many users (including me) sleep more deeply when supplementing with it. ZMA should not be taken with foods or supplements containing calcium because calcium blocks the absorption of zinc.

Dosage: As directed by manufacturer, generally 30–60 minutes before bedtime and on an empty stomach.

HYDRATION

Water is fundamental to health and well-being, so my message to you is to drink more of it. Being well hydrated reduces the likelihood of muscular injury, illness and fatigue, and plays an essential role in achieving your training goals.

Drinking 500ml–2 litres of water upon waking is a great way to rehydrate, and I strongly recommend you take a large bottle of water to work so that you can keep hydrated during the day. If I fail to do this, I definitely notice that I'm not as alert or energetic. Even being slightly dehydrated can have an adverse effect on your aerobic capacity. It's a good idea to mark lines on the bottle to show how much you should have drunk by certain times. If you are super-busy, drinking water and hydrating can become secondary to whatever else you're doing. You only notice once you are thirsty, which is too late. For this reason, I suggest you use the MyFitnessPal app to track your water intake, making a note of the number of cups or bottles you are consuming.

I recommend you keep to water as your main source of hydration. If that gets boring, try adding some fresh lemon juice. Apart from adding flavour, it helps to keep your blood sugar stable. I always try to start my day with 2 litres of water to which I add Precision electrolyte tablets containing sodium, calcium, potassium, phosphate and magnesium. I try to finish the entire 2 litres before I leave for training. If this isn't for you, I suggest you at the very least use some BCAAs (see page 214).

HYDRATION TIPS

» **Aim to drink** a minimum of 2–5 litres of water a day.

» **Soft drinks,** including diet versions, offer nothing in the way of good nutrition – they are simply full of sweetness – so it's best to avoid them. This is certainly true if you are looking to lose weight. If going 'cold turkey' is just too difficult, limit your intake to a maximum of one can a day of the diet variety.

» **Use energy drinks very sparingly** and only when genuinely in need of an energy boost, such as pre-workout, during and surrounding training, or to keep you awake when desperately trying to finish your coursework or dissertation! Energy drinks are full of sugar and sometimes caffeine, so they are not great for you, and all those empty calories have to be factored into your daily macros. I would suggest you reach for the sugar free variety.

» **Tea and coffee** (without milk and sugar) are both fine to consume in moderation, but the caffeine content means you should try to limit yourself to three cups a day. You would be shocked to know how much sugar and fat goes into some of our most popular beverages. A caramel latte, for example, is a sugar nightmare.

HOW DO I KNOW IF I AM HYDRATED?

The answer to this question is really simple: just look at the colour of your pee. If it's pale, you are hydrated and ready to go. If it's dark, you are dehydrated and need to drink. If you want further confirmation, compare the colour against the chart below.

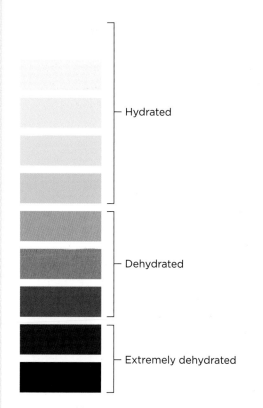

It's really important to check your urine before beginning to exercise, whether that's a session in the gym, an easy jog, getting ready for a race, or taking part in a match. Exercising properly involves losing fluid through perspiration, so make sure you have plenty to lose in the first place.

ALCOHOL

I must start by dispelling the idea that rugby encourages a macho culture that thinks drinking is 'cool' and makes you a 'real' man. Among professional rugby players that could not be further from the truth. Having the odd beer in a team-bonding session is fine, but on the whole, all the players I know will go months and months without drinking. The reasons are simple:

>> Getting drunk puts you at risk of injury, which can bring your career to an abrupt halt.

>> Hangovers make training and eating difficult, and ultimately affect your results.

>> The calories from alcohol have no nutritional value, so it is wasteful to put them into your body.

>> When combined with carbohydrates, fats and proteins, alcohol is the first fuel to be used, so it delays the fat-burning process and contributes to greater fat storage.

>> The body breaks down alcohol as sugars, so if you aren't very good at dealing with sugars (overweight people are in this camp), you will just store them as fat.

The alcohol in booze is a chemical called ethanol, which contains 7 calories per gram. It can't be stored in the body, so it is treated like a poison and broken down to get rid of it. This happens in the liver, but the liver can process only a percentage of the alcohol, so the excess calories are stored as fat.

I've often seen people drop loads of weight when they get on top of their booze habits. In fact, drinking alcohol can in some cases be the biggest factor limiting fat loss.

Here is my view on alcohol. If you are a big drinker, there is no point my telling you to stop. What I do suggest is that you try to cut down to a very limited amount, and to change what you drink. This is not only going to help you with this training programme, but with life in your general. However I know it is easier said than done, so here are some ideas for cutting back.

If you are a huge beer drinker, change to something like vodka with fresh lime and soda, and sip it rather than neck it down. A white wine spritzer is also a good alternative. This will reduce the overall number of calories that you are taking into your body.

If you are in the habit of drinking a glass or two of wine with dinner on weekdays and going big at the weekend, try to cut down by drinking only at the weekend. It's a good start, and is even better if you have a glass of water between every alcoholic drink.

TRY TO CUT ALCOHOL DOWN TO A LIMITED AMOUNT AND CHANGE WHAT YOU DRINK

Chapter 7
RECIPES

Anyone who knows me would not describe me as a masterchef. I lack that creative spark, but I can cook and I can follow a recipe. My amazing girlfriend cooks all the meals at home, which makes my life easier, and she makes them must tastier than I do.

When I cook, I tend to do a big piece of protein, a pile of carbs and loads of veg, basically because I'm usually pushed for time. At one low point in my culinary past, I lived on cold white fish, brown rice and broccoli amongst other things for 6 months, which was as grim as it sounds. It got me amazing results, but I don't recommend you eat like that. I want you to enjoy what you eat and to understand that healthy eating doesn't have to be boring.

My quest for good flavoursome food led me to team up with **Omar Meziane**, whom I first met when he was cooking for the Wasps rugby team. Wasps used to train at some of the worst training facilities in the premiership, and the only highlight of being there was Omar's cooking. We players might have spent the morning bogged down in something resembling a farmer's field that was masquerading as a rugby pitch, but Omar's food would always put a smile on our faces.

Omar is a professional chef who worked in restaurants and hotels before deciding to move into professional sport. Apart from Wasps, he has also worked with other teams, including England Cricket, England Rugby, Southampton FC, Northampton Saints and Team GB. He is dedicated to getting the very best from everyday ingredients, and he constantly demonstrates that simple, nutritious meals can be delicious and exciting.

Having made a number of recipe videos with Omar in the past, which you can see on my website and at www.youtube.com/thejameshaskell, I knew there was no better person to work when compiling this section of the book. If you want to know more about Omar please follow him on social media @TweatFresh.

The recipes are split into those with carbohydrates and those without. They are all super-healthy and full of flavour. Once you have worked out your calorie and macro counts (see page 201), you can take any of these recipes and edit the listed ingredients according to your needs. For example, if you are building muscle, you will need to increase things to hit your daily macros. That's where using an app like MyFitnessPal can be useful: it will give you a good idea of how much protein, fat and carbohydrate you need, and record the amounts you had at your previous meal.

Note: If you are allergic to an ingredient, or just don't like it, simply replace it with something of equal nutritional value. For example, if you can't have dairy, go for almond milk; if you can't eat fish, opt for chicken.

KITCHEN ESSENTIALS

You don't have to go mad and buy everything at once, but getting some essentials is key.

›› Good-quality pots and pans. I would choose heavy-based items – a non-stick frying pan, a wok and a selection of saucepans.

›› Airtight plastic containers. These are incredibly useful when you prepare food in advance. You will be using them throughout the plan, so buy a dozen or more, making sure they are large enough to hold your usual meal size.

›› Decent knives. You'll be doing a lot of food preparation, so having sharp, well-balanced knives will make that activity a lot easier. Blunt knives are frustrating and dangerous – far more likely to slip when you are cutting and cause a nasty injury. In my experience, all you need is a 20cm chef's knife, a small paring knife and a bread knife. You don't have to buy the most expensive. Handle them and see what feels right in your hand. Apart from that, make sure they are robust, easy to clean and resistant to rust.

›› Kitchen scales. As tracking your food is an essential element of following the programmes in this book, it's important to have some reliable scales to hand. I find digital ones are the best.

STORE-CUPBOARD ESSENTIALS

Now you have got rid of all the bad food in your house, it's important to stock up with what you need. Being prepared will make your life so much easier. Here are some food items that it's always worth having in your cupboards, fridge or freezer.

›› Asparagus
›› Broccoli
›› Brown rice
›› Chicken breasts
›› Chilli powder or flakes
›› Coconut oil – although oftened condemned for being high in saturated fat, I really like to cook with this as it's a great energy source. Use in moderation.
›› Eggs
›› Garlic
›› Honey
›› Lemons
›› Olive oil
›› Porridge oats
›› Rapeseed oil
›› Reduced sodium soy sauce
›› Salt and pepper
›› Steak
›› Sweet potato
›› Whey protein powder

COOK'S NOTES

Unless stated otherwise within the recipes:
›› **All spoon measures are level.**
›› **All eggs are medium.**
›› **All fruit and vegetables are medium.**
›› **Onions and garlic should be peeled before use.**

HAM, FETA & FIG FLATBREAD

SERVES 1

2 tbsp cottage cheese
1 wholemeal pitta bread
1–2 slices of Parma ham
2 ripe fresh figs, sliced
2 tbsp crumbled feta cheese

Energy (kCal) 349/serving	
Fat (g) 11	Fibre (g) 6.5
Sat fat (g) 6	Protein (g) 20
Carbs (g) 39	Salt (g) 2.3
Sugar (g) 10	

1 Preheat the grill until medium hot.

2 Spread the cottage cheese over one side of the pitta bread (do not split the bread open). Tear the ham into big pieces and place over the cottage cheese.

3 Place the fig slices over the ham. Sprinkle the feta on the top and pop under the grill.

4 Grill until the feta starts to brown and serve immediately.

Prep: 5 minutes / Cook: 5 minutes / Skill: simple

ALMOND FRENCH TOAST

SERVES 1

2 eggs
2 slices of brioche
1 tbsp ground almonds
1–2 tsp coconut oil
2 tbsp Greek yoghurt
100g mixed fresh berries
1 tbsp runny honey

Energy (kCal) 678/serving	
Fat (g) 33	Fibre (g) 4
Sat fat (g) 13	Protein (g) 29
Carbs (g) 64	Salt (g) 1.1
Sugar (g) 32	

1 Crack the eggs into a bowl and whisk well.

2 Heat a sauté pan over a medium heat.

3 Quickly dip the brioche slices into the eggs, then sprinkle both sides with the ground almonds.

4 Put the coconut oil into the pan, swirl it around, then add the brioche. Cook for 1–2 minutes on each side, or until golden brown. Transfer to a serving plate.

5 Spoon the yoghurt and berries on top, and drizzle over the honey before serving.

Prep: 5 minutes / Cook: 2–3 minutes / Skill: simple

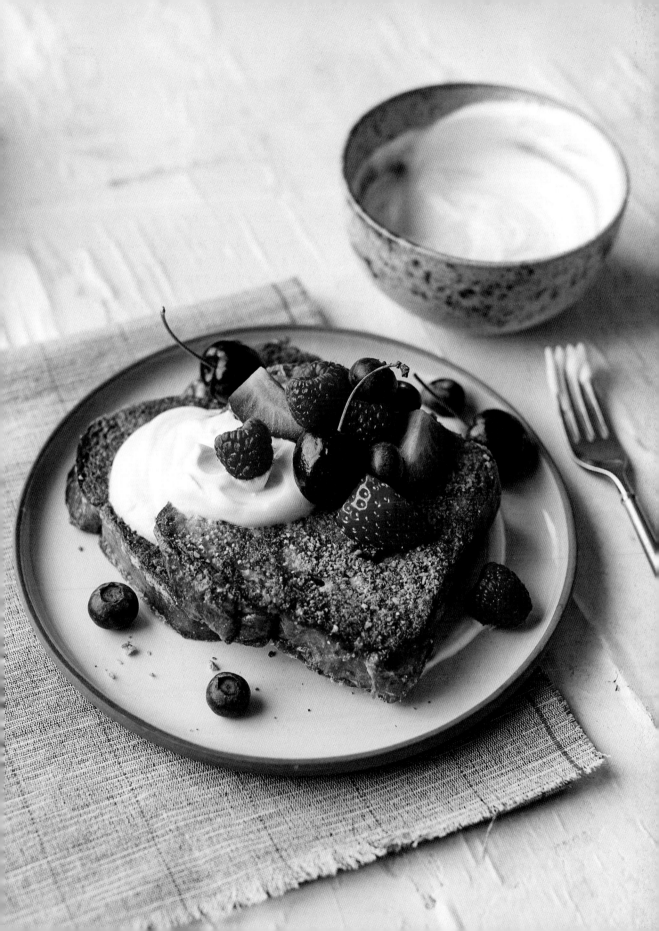

CRUSHED PEAS & AVOCADO WITH CHILLI ON SOURDOUGH TOAST

SERVES 1

100g fresh or defrosted
frozen peas
½ ripe avocado,
roughly chopped
¼ red chilli, finely chopped
juice of ½ lime
4–5 mint leaves, finely chopped
1 thick slice of sourdough bread
salt and pepper

Energy (kCal) 370/serving	
Fat (g) 17	Fibre (g) 10
Sat fat (g) 3.5	Protein (g) 13
Carbs (g) 35	Salt (g) 0.5
Sugar (g) 4	

1 Preheat the grill until medium hot.

2 Cook the peas for 1 minute in boiling water. Drain and place in a bowl.

3 Add the avocado and chilli to the peas and use a fork to lightly crush them together. Fold in the lime juice and mint, then season to taste with salt and pepper.

4 Toast the sourdough, spoon the avocado mixture over it and serve.

Prep: 10 minutes / Cook: 1 minute / Skill: simple

CORN & CHILLI FRITTERS

SERVES 1

1 spring onion, finely chopped
¼ red chilli, finely chopped
1 small bunch of coriander,
finely chopped
2 tbsp cooked kidney beans
100g frozen or tinned
sweetcorn
1 egg
25g plain flour
50ml semi-skimmed milk
1 tbsp olive oil

Energy (kCal) 400/serving	
Fat (g) 20	Fibre (g) 6
Sat fat (g) 4	Protein (g) 17
Carbs (g) 35	Salt (g) 0.3
Sugar (g) 5.5	

1 Place the spring onion, chilli and coriander in a bowl. Add the kidney beans and corn and stir well.

2 Crack the egg into a separate bowl, add the flour and milk and mix well to form a thick batter.

3 Add the sweetcorn mixture to the batter and stir until all the ingredients are well coated.

4 Heat a sauté pan over a medium heat. Add the olive oil, swirl it around, then place spoonfuls of the batter in the pan to make 2 medium-sized fritters. Cook for 1–2 minutes on each side and serve.

Prep: 10 minutes / Cook: 10 minute / Skill: simple

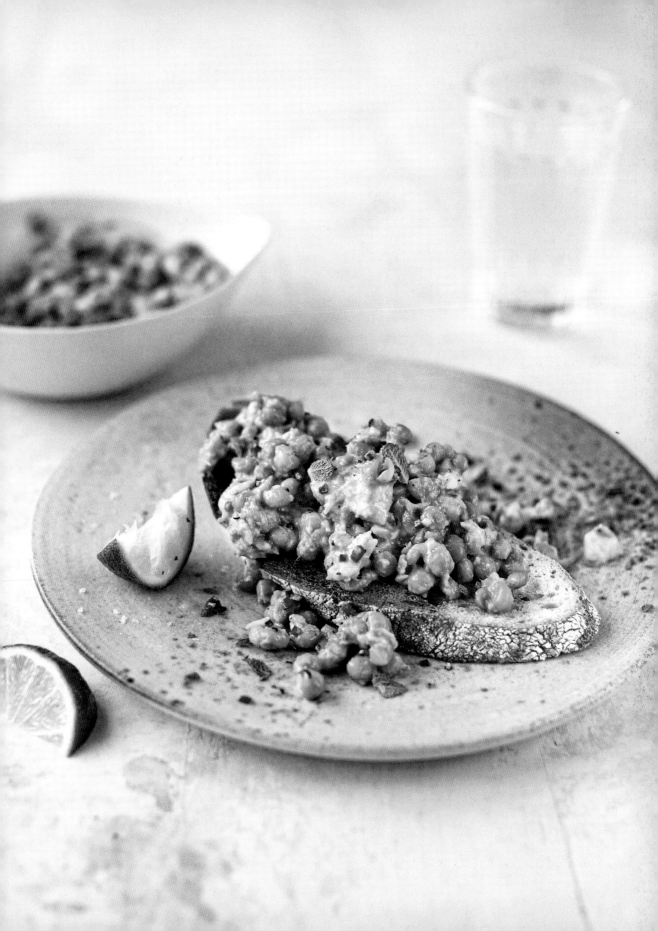

SCRAMBLED EGGS WITH CHORIZO & SWEET POTATO HASH

SERVES 1

1 small sweet potato
75g cooked mixed beans
40g chorizo, roughly chopped
2 eggs
1 knob of butter
15g feta cheese
salt and pepper

Energy (kCal) 633/serving	
Fat (g) 29	Fibre (g) 10
Sat fat (g) 11	Protein (g) 36
Carbs (g) 48	Salt (g) 2.6
Sugar (g) 11.5	

1 Preheat the oven to 180°C/Fan 160°C/Gas 4. Line a baking tray with baking parchment.

2 Wrap the sweet potato in foil and place in the oven for 15–20 minutes, or until soft to the touch. Remove the foil, slice the potato down the middle and gently peel away the skin. Allow the flesh to cool, then chop it into 2cm dice. Transfer to a heatproof bowl and mix in the beans.

3 Roughly chop the chorizo, place it on the prepared baking tray and put into the oven for 5 minutes. Add it to the bowl of sweet potato and stir to combine. Return the mixture to the baking tray and pop back into the oven for 5 minutes, or until warmed through.

4 Crack the eggs into a saucepan, season with salt and pepper and whisk together. Add the knob of butter and cook the eggs, stirring constantly, until scrambled.

5 To serve, place the hash on a plate, top with the scrambled eggs and crumble the feta cheese over the top.

Prep: 10 minutes / Cook: 30 minutes / Skill: simple

BLENDED FRUIT BOWL

SERVES 1

170g frozen mixed berries
1 small banana
4 tbsp almond milk
3 tbsp blueberries
1–2 tsp flaxseeds
1 tbsp almonds, roughly
  chopped

Energy (kCal) 281/serving	
Fat (g) 12	Fibre (g) 9
Sat fat (g) 1	Protein (g) 8
Carbs (g) 31	Salt (g) Trace
Sugar (g) 29	

1 Place the berries, banana and almond milk in a food processor and blend until smooth.

2 Pour the mixture into a serving bowl and sprinkle over the remaining ingredients.

Prep: 5 minutes / Skill: simple

COCONUT PORRIDGE

SERVES 1

50g porridge oats
100ml reduced-fat
    coconut milk
125ml almond milk
1 tsp coconut oil
1 tsp runny honey
1 tsp almond butter
1 tsp omega seeds (a blend of
    seeds high in omega-3 fats)

Energy (kCal) 405/serving	
Fat (g) 21	Fibre (g) 5
Sat fat (g) 10	Protein (g) 9
Carbs (g) 42	Salt (g) 0.2
Sugar (g) 11	

1 Put the oats, coconut milk, almond milk and coconut oil into a saucepan and place on a medium heat. Cook, stirring often, for 7–8 minutes, or until the mixture has thickened into a porridge.

2 Pour the porridge into a bowl. Drizzle over the honey, dot the almond butter on top and sprinkle with the omega seeds.

Prep: 1 minute / Cook: 7–8 minutes / Skill: simple

EGGS WITH YOGHURT, FLATBREAD, NUTS & SEEDS

SERVES 1

1 garlic clove, finely chopped
2 tbsp Greek yoghurt
juice of ½ lemon
2 eggs
½ tsp smoked paprika
pinch of dried chilli flakes
1 tbsp omega seeds
salt and pepper
1 warmed pitta bread, to serve

Energy (kCal) 495/serving	
Fat (g) 24	Fibre (g) 3
Sat fat (g) 7	Protein (g) 28
Carbs (g) 41	Salt (g) 1.3
Sugar (g) 3.5	

1 Place the garlic in a bowl. Add the yoghurt plus some salt and pepper and stir to combine.

2 Bring a shallow pan of water to the boil and add the lemon juice. Crack an egg into a cup, then slide it into the water. Repeat with the other egg. Poach for about 4 minutes, until the white is set but the yolk is still soft. Remove the eggs with a slotted spoon, and place the spoon over kitchen paper to absorb excess water.

3 Spoon the yoghurt mixture into a serving bowl, place the poached eggs on top and sprinkle over the smoked paprika, chilli flakes and omega seeds. Serve with the warm pitta bread.

Prep: 10 minutes / Cook: 5 minutes / Skill: moderate

PECAN & ALMOND GRANOLA

SERVES 8

100g dates, pitted
200g porridge oats
100g flaked almonds
50g pecan nuts,
    roughly chopped
20g pumpkin seeds
4 tbsp runny honey
4 tbsp coconut oil
Greek yoghurt, to serve

Energy (kCal) 327/serving	
Fat (g) 20	Fibre (g) 3
Sat fat (g) 6	Protein (g) 7.5
Carbs (g) 27.5	Salt (g) Trace
Sugar (g) 12	

1 Preheat the oven to 160°C/Fan 140°C/Gas 3.

2 Put the dates into a small saucepan and add just enough water to cover them. Place over a medium heat and allow to simmer for 10 minutes, or until very soft. Transfer to a food processor and blend until smooth.

3 Combine all the remaining ingredients, apart from the yoghurt, in a large bowl. Pour in the puréed dates and stir well.

4 Spread the mixture out evenly on a baking tray and bake for 30 minutes, or until the mixture is dry and crisp. Allow to cool before storing in an airtight jar for up to 2 weeks. Alternatively, eat straight away with a large spoonful of Greek yoghurt.

Prep: 5 minutes / Cook: 40 minutes / Skill: simple

PROTEIN PANCAKES

SERVES 1

2 scoops porridge oats
1 scoop whey protein powder
pinch of ground cinnamon
1 egg
1 tbsp milk
1 tbsp coconut oil

To serve

fruit, nuts, honey, peanut
    butter, or as you wish

Energy (kCal) 476/serving	
Fat (g) 22	Fibre (g) 4
Sat fat (g) 13	Protein (g) 33
Carbs (g) 34	Salt (g) 0.2
Sugar (g) 1	

1 Pop the oats into a food processor and blend to a flour.

2 Transfer to a large bowl, add all the remaining ingredients except the coconut oil, and whisk until you have a batter. Cover and leave to rest in the fridge for 15 minutes.

3 Heat a sauté pan over a medium heat. Add the coconut oil, swirl it around the pan, then spoon in the batter to make 4 pancakes. Cook for 2 minutes on each side.

4 Serve the pancakes with your favourite toppings. Mine are peanut butter, manuka honey, bananas and blueberries.

Prep: 5 minutes + 15 minutes resting / Cook: 5 minutes / Skill: simple

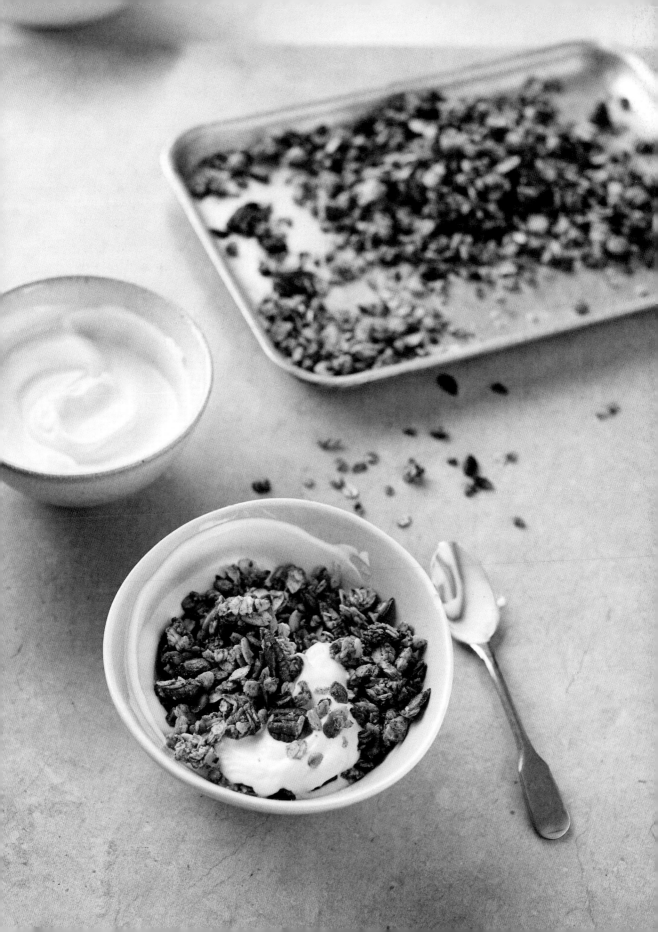

STEAK WITH EGGS & WATERCRESS SAUCE

SERVES 1

juice of ½ lemon
2 eggs
1 x 175g sirloin steak
1 tbsp olive oil

For the watercress sauce
¼ red chilli, deseeded
1 bunch of watercress
1 tbsp olive oil
1 tbsp white wine vinegar
2 tbsp water
salt and pepper

Energy (kCal) 614/serving	
Fat (g) 42	Fibre (g) 1.5
Sat fat (g) 10	Protein (g) 59
Carbs (g) 0	Salt (g) 0.9
Sugar (g) 0	

1 First make the sauce: place all the ingredients for it in a food processor and blend until smooth. Taste and adjust the seasoning.

2 Meanwhile, heat a frying pan over a high heat. Season the steak and rub the olive oil into it on both sides. Place in the pan and cook for 2–3 minutes on each side.

3 Bring a shallow pan of water to the boil and add the lemon juice. Crack an egg into a cup, then slide it into the water. Repeat with the other egg. Poach for about 4 minutes, until the white is set but the yolk is still soft.

4 Slice the steak and arrange on a serving plate. Pour the sauce over the meat and serve with the poached eggs.

Prep: 10 minutes / Cook: 10 minutes / Skill: moderate

ROASTED TOMATOES, SCRAMBLED EGGS & PARMESAN

SERVES 1

2 plum tomatoes, halved
leaves from 1 sprig of thyme
3 eggs
knob of butter
freshly grated Parmesan
    cheese, to taste
1 tbsp cottage cheese
salt and pepper

Energy (kCal) 375/serving	
Fat (g) 25	Fibre (g) 2.5
Sat fat (g) 10	Protein (g) 25
Carbs (g) 8	Salt (g) 1
Sugar (g) 8	

1 Preheat the grill until very hot.

2 Place the tomatoes on a baking tray. Season with salt and pepper, then sprinkle with the thyme. Cook under the grill for 2–3 minutes, or until browned.

3 Crack the eggs into a saucepan, season with salt and pepper, and whisk together. Add the knob of butter and cook the eggs over a medium heat, stirring constantly, until scrambled. Transfer to a plate and grate over as much Parmesan as you fancy.

4 Serve the eggs with the tomatoes and cottage cheese alongside.

Prep: 5 minutes / Cook: 10 minutes / Skill: simple

TURKEY ESCALOPE WITH 'CHIMICHURRI' SAUCE

SERVES 1

1 x 175g turkey escalope

For the sauce
1 garlic clove
large handful of baby
    spinach leaves
pinch of dried chilli flakes
3 tbsp olive oil
2 tbsp white wine vinegar
salt and pepper

Energy (kCal) 480/serving	
Fat (g) 35	Fibre (g) 0.5
Sat fat (g) 5	Protein (g) 44
Carbs (g) 0	Salt (g) 0.3
Sugar (g) 0	

1 Preheat the grill until medium hot.

2 Place all the sauce ingredients in a food processor and blend until smooth. Check the seasoning and set aside.

3 Season the turkey with salt and pepper, then pop under the grill and cook for 3–4 minutes on each side, until cooked through.

4 Serve the turkey with the sauce poured over it. This breakfast goes really well with eggs, so add some if you want to increase the protein.

Prep: 10 minutes / Cook: 8 minutes / Skill: simple

MUSHROOMS WITH SPINACH & SCRAMBLED EGGS

SERVES 1

10g of butter
2 handfuls of mushrooms
   (oyster, chestnut, button,
   or whatever you fancy)
juice of ½ lemon
2 handfuls of baby
   spinach leaves
3 eggs
1 tsp pumpkin seeds
salt and pepper

Energy (kCal) 382/serving	
Fat (g) 29	Fibre (g) 2
Sat fat (g) 10	Protein (g) 30
Carbs (g) 1	Salt (g) 1
Sugar (g) 0.5	

1 Heat a sauté pan over a high heat. Add 2 knobs of the butter and the mushrooms, season with salt and pepper, and cook for 5–6 minutes, until lightly browned.

2 Add the lemon juice followed by the spinach. Once the spinach has wilted, remove the pan from the heat.

3 Crack the eggs into a saucepan, season with salt and pepper and whisk together. Add the remaining knob of butter and cook the eggs over a medium heat, stirring constantly, until scrambled.

4 Serve the eggs alongside the mushroom and spinach mixture, with the pumpkin seeds sprinkled on top.

Prep: 10 minutes / Cook: 10–12 minutes / Skill: simple

SALMON, EGG, WATERCRESS & HAM MUFFINS

SERVES 1

2–3 slices of Parma ham
handful of watercress
2 eggs
pinch of dried chilli flakes
2 slices of smoked salmon
salt and pepper

Energy (kCal) 285/serving	
Fat (g) 18	Fibre (g) 0
Sat fat (g) 5	Protein (g) 31
Carbs (g) 0.8	Salt (g) 2.7
Sugar (g) 0.8	

1 Preheat the oven to 180°C/Fan 160°C/Gas 4.

2 Line two of the cups in a non-stick muffin tin with the Parma ham. Divide the watercress between the two.

3 Crack the eggs into a bowl. Add the chilli flakes plus some salt and pepper, and beat together with a fork.

4 Pour the eggs over the watercress. Top each cup with half the salmon, then bake for 10 minutes, or until the eggs are cooked.

Prep: 10 minutes / Cook: 10 minutes / Skill: simple

ROASTED SALMON WITH SPINACH, AVOCADO & OMEGA SEEDS

SERVES 1

1 x 125g fillet of salmon
knob of butter
2–3 large handfuls of
    baby spinach leaves
½ small ripe avocado,
    coarsely chopped
juice of ½ lemon
1 tsp omega seeds
salt and pepper

Energy (kCal) 475/serving	
Fat (g) 37	Fibre (g) 4
Sat fat (g) 9	Protein (g) 30
Carbs (g) 2	Salt (g) 0.3
Sugar (g) 0.5	

1 Preheat the oven to 200°C/Fan 180°C/Gas 6.

2 Place the salmon in a roasting tray and season with salt and pepper. Roast in the oven for 7–8 minutes.

3 Meanwhile, heat a saucepan over a high heat, then add the butter, spinach and some seasoning. Cook the spinach until it has wilted, then drain well and place in a bowl.

4 Add the avocado and lemon juice to the spinach and stir gently to combine.

5 Serve the salmon with the spinach mixture, and sprinkle the omega seeds over the top.

Prep: 10 minutes / Cook: 10 minutes / Skill: simple

SPINACH PESTO WITH GRILLED MACKEREL

SERVES 1

handful of baby spinach leaves
small bunch of basil
1 tsp ground almonds
2 tsp freshly grated
    Parmesan cheese
1 tbsp olive oil
1 garlic clove
2 fresh mackerel fillets,
    about 60g each
½ lemon
salt and pepper
2 small eggs

Energy (kCal) 588/serving	
Fat (g) 47	Fibre (g) 0.2
Sat fat (g) 11	Protein (g) 40
Carbs (g) 0.5	Salt (g) 0.9
Sugar (g) 0.3	

1 Preheat the grill until hot.

2 Meanwhile, place the spinach, basil, ground almonds, Parmesan, olive oil and garlic in a food processor and blend until you have a smooth pesto. Set aside.

3 Place the mackerel in a grill tray, flesh side down. Season with salt and pepper, then place under the grill and cook for 2 minutes on each side.

4 Spread the pesto over the skin side of the fish and serve with a squeeze of lemon juice. This is great with poached or scrambled eggs.

Prep: 10 minutes / Cook: 8 minutes / Skill: simple

AVOCADO SALSA WITH POACHED EGGS

SERVES 1

½ ripe avocado,
    roughly chopped
¼ red onion, finely sliced
¼ red chilli, finely sliced
juice of 1 lime
1 small bunch of coriander,
    roughly chopped
2 plum tomatoes, diced
1 tbsp pumpkin seeds
juice of ½ lemon
2 eggs
salt and pepper

Energy (kCal) 460/serving	
Fat (g) 33	Fibre (g) 8
Sat fat (g) 7	Protein (g) 23
Carbs (g) 14.5	Salt (g) 0.5
Sugar (g) 11	

1 Place the avocado, onion and chilli in a large bowl. Pour in the lime juice, then add the coriander and tomatoes. Season with salt and pepper, add the pumpkin seeds and toss well. Set aside.

2 Bring a shallow pan of water to the boil and add the lemon juice. Crack an egg into a cup, then slide it into the water. Repeat with the other egg. Poach for about 4 minutes, until the white is set but the yolk is still soft.

3 Serve the eggs alongside the avocado salsa.

Prep: 10 minutes / Cook: 5 minutes / Skill: simple

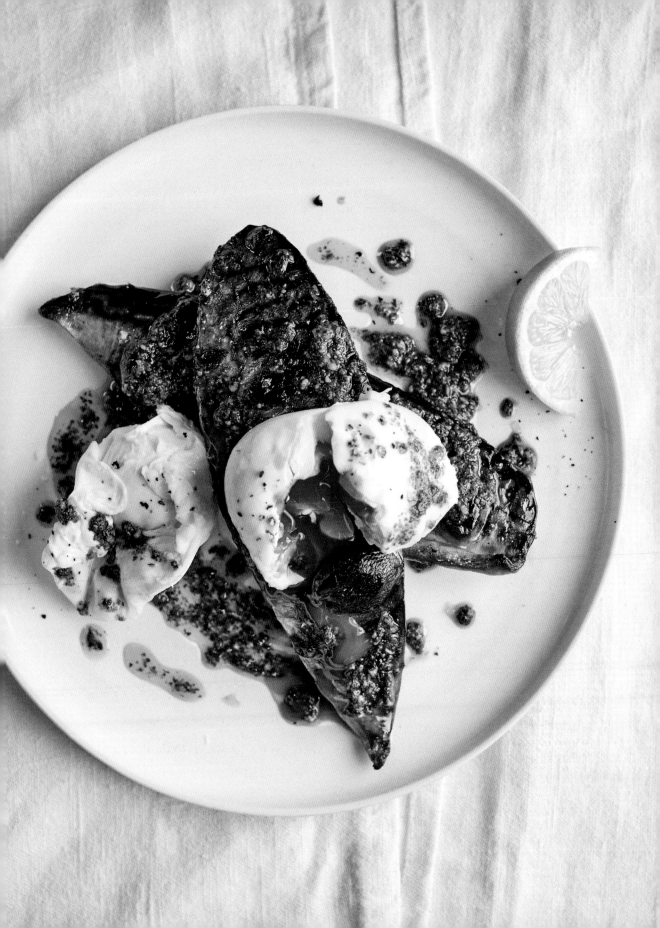

ROASTED PEACHES WITH PARMA HAM & ROSEMARY

SERVES 1

1 peach, halved and
    stone removed
leaves from 1 sprig of
    rosemary, roughly chopped
2 tsp runny honey
2 tbsp cottage cheese
2 slices of Parma ham

Energy (kCal) 150/serving	
Fat (g) 4.5	Fibre (g) 1
Sat fat (g) 2	Protein (g) 9
Carbs (g) 17	Salt (g) 1.2
Sugar (g) 17	

1 Preheat the grill until hot.

2 Place both halves of the peach on a grill tray. Sprinkle with the rosemary leaves, then drizzle with the honey. Pop under the grill for 3–4 minutes, or until the peach has caramelised and softened.

3 Spoon the cottage cheese into a serving bowl and place the peach halves on top. Drape the Parma ham over the peaches and serve.

Prep: 5 minutes / Cook: 5 minutes / Skill: simple

SMOKED SALMON & PEA OMELETTE

SERVES 1

3 eggs
50g smoked salmon,
    roughly chopped
50g fresh or frozen peas
1 tsp butter
1 tbsp ricotta cheese
salt and pepper

Energy (kCal) 438/serving	
Fat (g) 27	Fibre (g) 2.5
Sat fat (g) 9.5	Protein (g) 40
Carbs (g) 6	Salt (g) 2.3
Sugar (g) 1.5	

1 Preheat the grill until medium hot.

2 Crack the eggs into a bowl, season with salt and pepper and whisk together.

3 Place the salmon in a baking tray with the peas. Pop under the grill and gently warm through.

4 Place an omelette pan over a medium heat. Add the butter, swirl it around, then pour in the beaten eggs. Cook, swirling with the back of a fork until the underside is set and speckled brown, and the surface still looks creamy.

5 Take the pan off the heat and spread the ricotta over the omelette. Top with the salmon and peas, then roll it up and serve.

Prep: 10 minutes / Cook: 5 minutes / Skill: simple

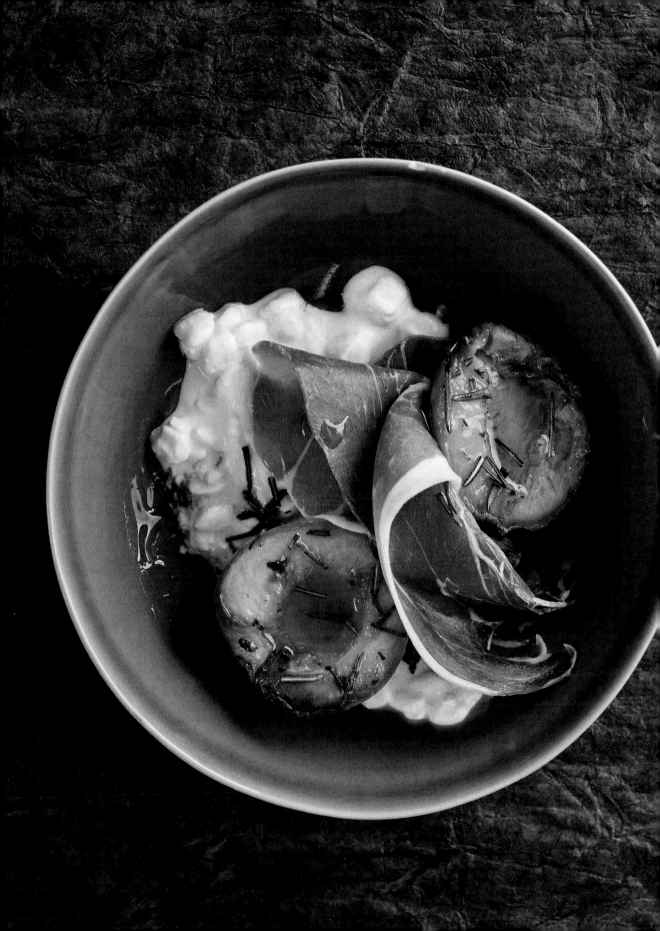

LUNCH HIGH-CARB LUNCH DISHES

These recipes have all been written so that each dish can be enjoyed hot and freshly cooked, or packed into a lidded plastic container and eaten on the go.

GRILLED CHICKEN WITH EDAMAME BEAN & CASHEW SALAD

SERVES 1

1 skinless chicken breast
75g brown rice
50g edamame beans
1 carrot, peeled and grated
juice of 1 lime
1 tsp honey
¼ red chilli, finely sliced
2 tsp dark soy sauce
25g cashew nuts
salt and pepper

Energy (kCal) 738/serving	
Fat (g) 19	Fibre (g) 10
Sat fat (g) 3.5	Protein (g) 54
Carbs (g) 82	Salt (g) 1.8
Sugar (g) 17	

1 Preheat the grill until very hot.

2 Slice the chicken breast lengthways into 4. Place on a grill tray and season with salt and pepper. Grill for 5–6 minutes on each side, or until cooked through. Set aside.

3 Place the rice in a saucepan, cover with water, add salt to taste and bring to the boil. Continue cooking for 20 minutes, or until the rice is cooked through. Drain and transfer to a serving bowl.

4 Meanwhile, bring a small saucepan of water to the boil, add the edamame beans and cook for 2–3 minutes. Drain well.

5 Arrange the beans and carrot on top of the rice.

6 Place the chicken in a separate bowl and pour the lime juice over it. Add the honey, chilli and soy sauce, toss well and place on top of the rice mixture. Sprinkle with the cashew nuts and serve.

Prep: 10 minutes / Cook: 30–40 minutes / Skill: simple

CURRIED BARLEY WITH ROASTED MACKEREL & CUMIN YOGHURT

SERVES 1

75g pearl barley
1 tbsp medium-hot
    curry powder
handful of baby spinach leaves
seeds from ½ pomegranate
1 tbsp walnut halves
2 fresh mackerel fillets,
    about 75g each
juice of ½ lemon
1 tsp ground cumin
1 tbsp Greek yoghurt
salt and pepper

Energy (kCal) 861/serving	
Fat (g) 43	Fibre (g) 9.5
Sat fat (g) 8	Protein (g) 41
Carbs (g) 73	Salt (g) 0.9
Sugar (g) 10	

1 Preheat the grill until very hot.

2 Place the barley in a saucepan, cover with water and add the curry powder and some seasoning. Bring to the boil, then simmer for 10–12 minutes, or until cooked through. Drain and place in a bowl. Fold in the baby spinach, the pomegranate seeds and walnuts. Season with salt and pepper, stir again and set aside.

3 Place the mackerel fillets, skin side up, on a grill tray and season with salt and pepper. Grill for 2 minutes on each side, then pour the lemon juice over the fish.

4 Place the barley mixture in a serving bowl and top with the mackerel. Stir the cumin into the yoghurt and spoon over the mackerel.

Prep: 10 minutes / Cook: 15 minutes / Skill: simple

HALLOUMI WITH MIXED BEANS & POMEGRANATE

SERVES 1

75g brown rice
50g cooked butterbeans
50g cooked kidney beans
handful of baby spinach leaves
seeds from ½ pomegranate
2 tbsp olive oil
2 slices of halloumi cheese,
    1.5cm thick, about 40g
    in total
2 tbsp hummus

Energy (kCal) 857/serving	
Fat (g) 43	Fibre (g) 15
Sat fat (g) 10	Protein (g) 25
Carbs (g) 85	Salt (g) 1.3
Sugar (g) 10	

1 Place the rice in a saucepan, cover with water and bring to the boil. Cook for 20–25 minutes, or until done. Drain and set aside.

2 Place the butterbeans and kidney beans in a bowl. Add the spinach and pomegranate seeds, then the rice and half the olive oil and toss well.

3 Heat a griddle pan until very hot. Brush the remaining olive oil over the halloumi and place in the griddle pan. Cook for 30 seconds on each side.

4 Place the hummus in a serving bowl and top with the rice and bean mixture. Sit the halloumi on top and serve.

Prep: 10 minutes / Cook: 25–30 minutes / Skill: simple

TURKEY KOFTAS WITH PERSIAN RICE

SERVES 1

200g minced turkey
½ tsp ground cumin
½ tsp ground cinnamon
pinch of ground coriander
salt and pepper

For the Persian rice

75g brown rice
2 tsp coconut oil
1 tbsp sultanas
4 dried apricots, chopped
1 tsp flaked almonds
1 tbsp dried cranberries
parsley, roughly chopped

Energy (kCal) 745/serving	
Fat (g) 19.5	Fibre (g) 0.6
Sat fat (g) 8.5	Protein (g) 60
Carbs (g) 85	Salt (g) 0.4
Sugar (g) 28	

1 Place the turkey in a large bowl and season with salt and pepper. Add the spices and mix gently until well combined. Divide the mixture into 4–6 equal pieces and roll each one into a cigar shape. Transfer to a plate and place in the fridge for 30 minutes.

2 Preheat the oven to 180°C/Fan 160°C/Gas 4.

3 Put the rice into a saucepan and cover with water. Bring to the boil and cook for 20–25 minutes, or until cooked through. Drain and place in a large bowl. Add the remaining ingredients and mix well. Cover and set aside.

4 Place the turkey koftas in a roasting tray and cook in the oven for 10 minutes, or until cooked through.

5 Place the rice mixture in a serving bowl, sit the koftas on top and serve.

**Prep: 15 minutes + 30 minutes chilling /
Cook: 25–30 minutes / Skill: simple**

ROAST SALMON SALAD

SERVES 1

3–4 new potatoes
½ ripe avocado,
    roughly chopped
1 tomato, diced
50g cooked kidney beans
50g cooked chickpeas
1 tbsp omega seeds
juice of 1 lemon
1 salmon fillet
salt and pepper

Energy (kCal) 709/serving	
Fat (g) 40	Fibre (g) 16
Sat fat (g) 8	Protein (g) 35
Carbs (g) 43	Salt (g) 0.14
Sugar (g) 6	

1 Preheat the oven to 200°C/Fan 180°C/Gas 6.

2 Place the potatoes in a small saucepan and cover with water. Bring to the boil and cook for 15–20 minutes, or until tender. Drain in a colander, then leave to cool. Shake off any excess water and cut the potatoes in half. Place in a serving bowl.

3 Add the avocado and tomato to the potatoes, along with the kidney beans, chickpeas and omega seeds. Stir gently, then squeeze over half the lemon juice.

4 Place the salmon in a roasting tray and season with salt and pepper. Roast in the oven for 7–8 minutes. Put the salmon on top of the salad and squeeze over the remaining lemon juice.

Prep: 10 minutes / Cook: 30 minutes / Skill: simple

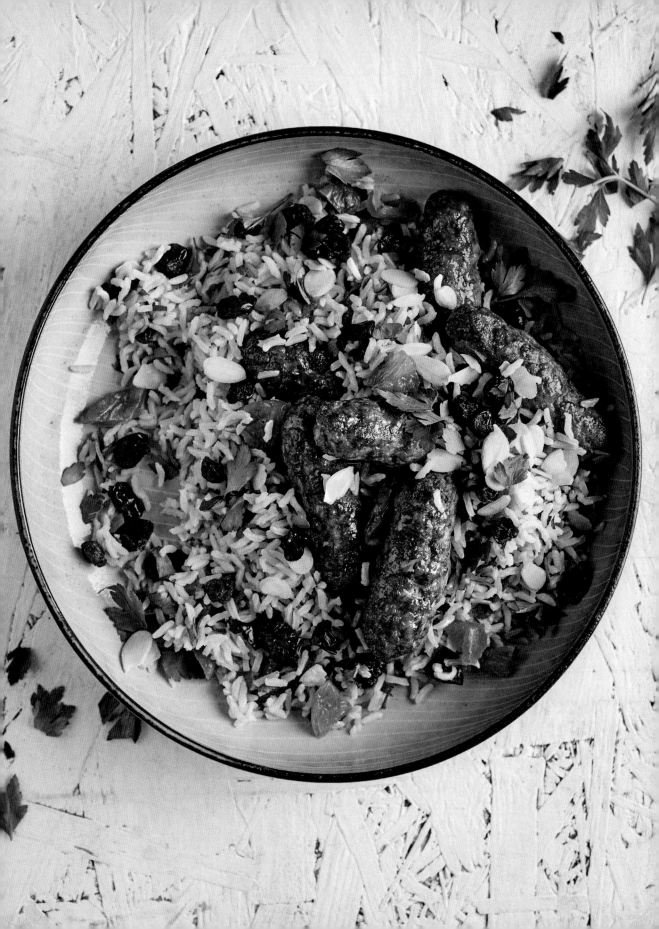

CHILLI & LIME CHICKEN WITH THAI NOODLE SALAD

SERVES 1

1 skinless chicken breast
½ red chilli, finely chopped
1 garlic clove, finely chopped
2 tsp runny honey
grated zest and juice of 1 lime

For the noodle salad

75g dried egg noodles
2 spring onions, finely chopped
5–6 mint leaves, finely chopped
1 garlic clove, finely chopped
¼ red chilli, finely chopped
2 tbsp roasted peanuts
2 tsp fish sauce

Energy (kCal) 656/serving	
Fat (g) 17	Fibre (g) 4.5
Sat fat (g) 3	Protein (g) 55
Carbs (g) 69	Salt (g) 3.8
Sugar (g) 16	

1 Slice the chicken breast lengthways into 4, then place in a bowl. Add the chilli, garlic, honey, lime zest and juice. Mix well, then cover the bowl and place in the fridge for 30 minutes.

2 Preheat the oven to 200°C/Fan 180°C/Gas 6.

3 Place the noodles in a saucepan, cover with water and bring to the boil. Cook for 4–5 minutes, or until soft. Drain, then rinse under running cold water. Shake off any excess water and pop the noodles into a large bowl.

4 Stir the spring onions, mint, garlic and chilli into the noodles. Add the peanuts and fish sauce and mix again.

5 Place the chicken in a roasting tray and pour the marinade over it. Cook in the oven for 8–10 minutes, or until cooked through.

6 Place the noodles in a serving bowl and top with the chicken. Pour any remaining sauce from the roasting tray over the meat.

**Prep: 15 minutes + 30 minutes chilling /
Cook: 15 minutes / Skill: simple**

TURKEY & BEETROOT MEATBALLS WITH PASTA SALAD

SERVES 1

2 small cooked beetroot,
  finely chopped
150g minced turkey
salt and pepper

For the salad

75g orzo pasta
small handful of parsley,
  finely chopped
50g cooked chickpeas
2 tbsp whole almonds
6 cherry tomatoes, halved
2 tsp olive oil

Energy (kCal) 880/serving	
Fat (g) 29	Fibre (g) 8.5
Sat fat (g) 3	Protein (g) 79
Carbs (g) 71	Salt (g) 0.5
Sugar (g) 10	

1 Place the beetroot in a bowl with the turkey. Season with salt and pepper and mix gently until well combined. Divide the mixture into 6–8 equal pieces and roll each one into a ball. Transfer to a plate and place in the fridge for 30 minutes.

2 Fill a small saucepan with water and add a pinch of salt. Bring to the boil, add the pasta and cook for 8 minutes, or until al dente. Drain, then cool by holding it under running cold water. Shake off any excess water and transfer to a clean bowl.

3 Add the parsley, chickpeas, almonds and tomatoes to the pasta.

4 Preheat the oven to 180°C/Fan 160°C/Gas 4.

5 Place the chilled meatballs in a roasting tray and cook in the oven for 7–8 minutes, or until cooked through.

6 Put the pasta salad into a serving bowl, top with the meatballs and serve.

Prep: 15 minutes + 30 minutes chilling / Cook: 15–20 minutes / Skill: simple

PORK & LIME CASHEW STIR-FRY

SERVES 1

75g brown rice
2 tsp coconut oil
150g pork tenderloin,
  sliced into thin rounds
1 carrot, peeled and finely
  sliced at an angle
2 spring onions, sliced
  at an angle
1 garlic clove, finely sliced
1 tbsp dark soy sauce
1 tbsp runny honey
½ tsp dried chilli flakes
handful of beansprouts
2 tbsp cashew nuts

Energy (kCal) 838/serving	
Fat (g) 30	Fibre (g) 9
Sat fat (g) 11	Protein (g) 49
Carbs (g) 90	Salt (g) 2.45
Sugar (g) 30	

1 Put the rice in a saucepan and cover with water. Bring to the boil and cook for 25–30 minutes, or until tender. Drain and set aside.

2 Heat a wok over a high heat and add the oil. Add the pork carefully and cook for 3–4 minutes, gently turning it now and then with a spatula. (Resist the temptation to shake the wok.)

3 Add the carrot, spring onions and garlic and continue cooking for 2–3 minutes, stirring only occasionally and never shaking the pan. Now add the soy sauce, honey and chilli flakes and cook for another 2 minutes. Lastly, add the beansprouts and cashew nuts and cook for a further 2 minutes.

4 Finally, add the rice to the wok and give everything a good toss. Serve in a large bowl.

Prep: 15 minutes / Cook: 30–35 minutes / Skill: simple

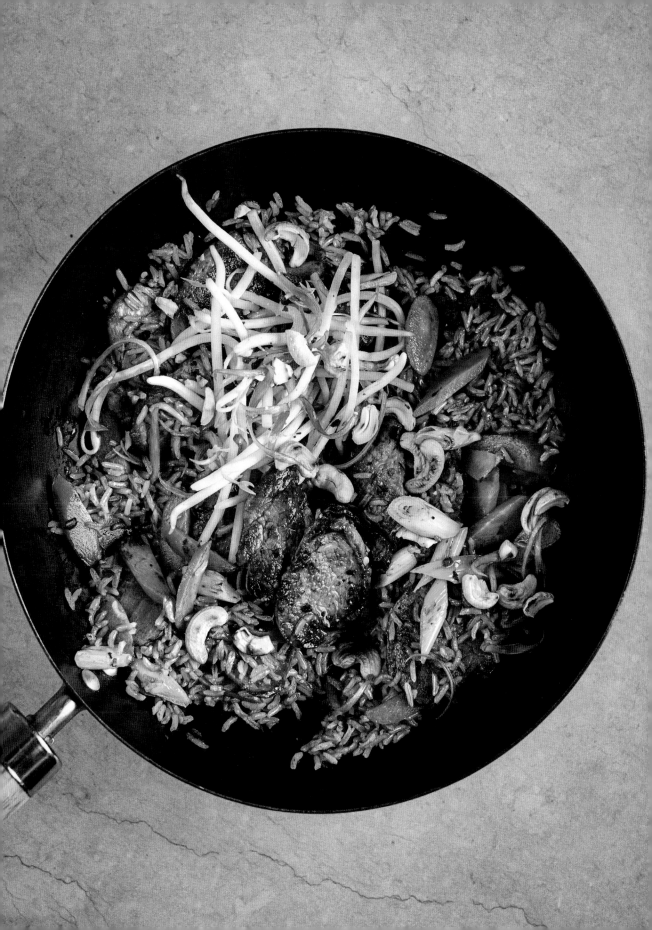

LAMB & HARISSA MEATBALLS WITH BULGUR WHEAT SALAD

150g lean minced lamb
2 tsp harissa paste
salt and pepper

For the salad
75g bulgur wheat
small handful of parsley,
    roughly chopped
4 mint leaves, roughly chopped
8 cherry tomatoes, halved
juice of ½ lemon
1 tbsp Greek yoghurt
salt and pepper

Energy (kCal) 650/serving	
Fat (g) 28	Fibre (g) 6
Sat fat (g) 13.5	Protein (g) 37
Carbs (g) 60	Salt (g) 0.2
Sugar (g) 5	

1 Place the lamb and harissa in a large bowl, season with salt and pepper, then stir gently to combine. Divide the mixture into 6–8 equal pieces and roll each one into a ball. Transfer to a plate and place in the fridge for 30 minutes.

2 Preheat the oven to 200°C/Fan 180°C/Gas 6.

3 Pour 150ml water into a saucepan and bring to the boil. Take off the heat, add the bulgur wheat and cover. Set aside for 20 minutes, or until the bulgur is fluffy and tender. Drain off any excess water and transfer the bulgur to a bowl.

4 Add the parsley, mint and tomatoes to the bulgur, then squeeze in the lemon juice. Stir well and season with salt and pepper.

5 Place the chilled meatballs in a roasting tray and roast for 8–10 minutes, or until cooked through.

6 To serve, place the salad in a serving bowl, top with the meatballs and yoghurt, and enjoy.

**Prep: 10 minutes + 30 minutes chilling /
Cook: 30–35 minutes / Skill: simple**

CHICKEN, CHORIZO, BUTTERBEAN & SWEET POTATO SALAD

SERVES 1

1 small sweet potato, unpeeled
6 mint leaves, finely chopped
75g cooked butterbeans
1 skinless chicken breast
50g chorizo, roughly chopped
juice of ½ lime
salt and pepper

Energy (kCal) 615/serving	
Fat (g) 19	Fibre (g) 11.5
Sat fat (g) 7	Protein (g) 55
Carbs (g) 51	Salt (g) 2.2
Sugar (g) 12	

1 Preheat the oven to 180°C/Fan 160°C/Gas 4.

2 Place the sweet potato in a roasting tray and bake in the oven for 30 minutes, or until soft to the touch. Allow to cool, then slice lengthways down the centre. Peel the skin away and cut the flesh into 6–8 chunks. Transfer to a large bowl.

3 Add the mint and butterbeans to the sweet potato and stir together gently.

4 Place the chicken breast in a roasting tray and season with salt and pepper. Roast in the oven for 15 minutes, or until cooked through. Allow to cool before slicing it into 6 pieces.

5 Place the chorizo in a roasting tray and cook in the oven for 5 minutes, just until it starts to brown and releases its fat. Add it to the sweet potato bowl.

6 To serve, place the chorizo mixture in a serving bowl and top with the chicken. Squeeze the lime juice over the chicken and enjoy.

Prep: 15 minutes / Cook: 45 minutes / Skill: simple

BEETROOT HUMMUS WITH VEGETABLES

SERVES 1

160g cooked chickpeas
200g cooked beetroot
juice of ½ lemon
2 garlic cloves
1 tbsp tahini
1 tsp ground cumin
4–5 tbsp olive oil
salt and pepper

Energy (kCal) 798/serving	
Fat (g) 57	Fibre (g) 15
Sat fat (g) 8	Protein (g) 19
Carbs (g) 43	Salt (g) 5
Sugar (g) 17.5	

1 Preheat the oven to 180°C/Fan 160°C/Gas 4.

2 Place all the ingredients for the hummus in a food processor and blend until smooth. Check the seasoning and set aside.

3 To serve, place 2–3 tablespoons of the hummus in a bowl and top with your choice of vegetables. Squeeze over the lemon juice and enjoy.

Prep: 10 minutes / Cook: 8–10 minutes / Skill: simple

CHILLI & SOY-GLAZED CHICKEN WITH BEAN SALAD

SERVES 1

1 skinless chicken breast
1 tsp runny honey
1 tbsp dark soy sauce
pinch of dried chilli flakes

For the salad
50g fresh or frozen peas
50g podded broad beans
2 spring onions, finely sliced
1 tbsp cashew nuts
1 tbsp toasted desiccated
   coconut

Energy (kCal) 349/serving	
Fat (g) 11	Fibre (g) 6.5
Sat fat (g) 6	Protein (g) 20
Carbs (g) 39	Salt (g) 2.3
Sugar (g) 10	

1 Preheat the oven to 180°C/Fan 160°C/Gas 4.

2 Place the chicken in a bowl with the honey, soy sauce and chilli flakes. Mix well and leave to marinate for 10 minutes. Transfer the chicken to a roasting tray and pour the marinade over it. Place in the oven for 12–15 minutes, or until cooked through. Allow to cool slightly before cutting into 6 slices.

3 To make the salad, cook the peas and beans in boiling salted water. Drain in a colander, then hold under running cold water until cool. Shake off the excess water. Add to a bowl with the remaining ingredients and toss well to combine. Serve on a plate with the chicken slices arranged on top.

**Prep: 10 minutes + 10 minutes marinating /
Cook: 12–15 minutes / Skill: simple**

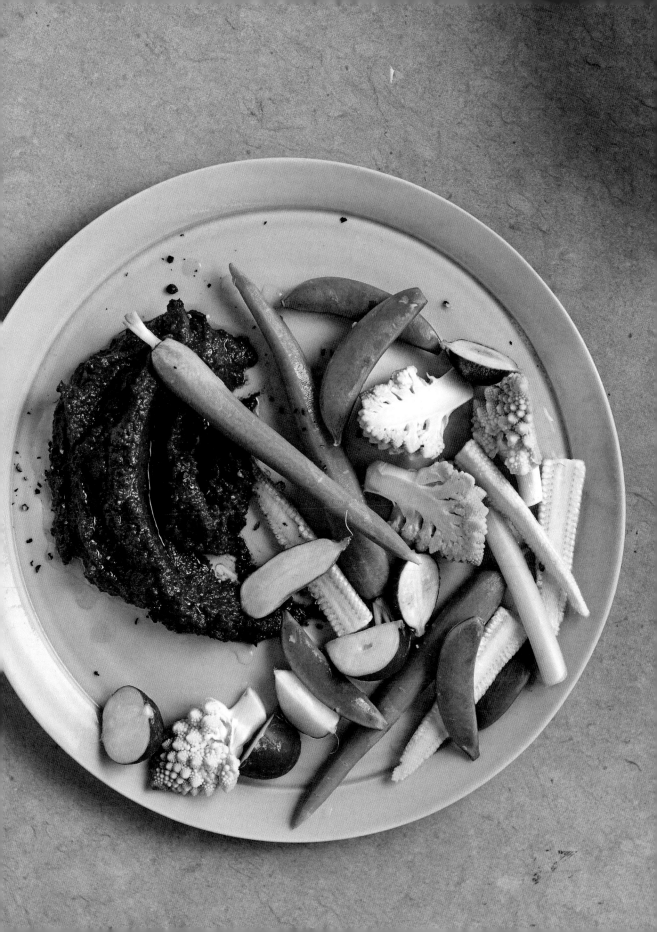

CRISPY VIETNAMESE BEEF WITH PEANUT SALAD

SERVES 1

1 x 150g fillet steak
1 tbsp cornflour
pinch of dried chilli flakes
1 tsp coconut oil
salt and pepper

For the salad

1 small wedge of red cabbage
    (100g), finely shredded
1 small carrot, peeled
    and grated
1 tbsp rice wine vinegar
    or white wine vinegar
small handful of fresh
    coriander, finely chopped
2 tbsp roasted peanuts
2 lime wedges

Energy (kCal) 503/serving	
Fat (g) 25	Fibre (g) 6
Sat fat (g) 9	Protein (g) 45
Carbs (g) 21	Salt (g) 0.4
Sugar (g) 10	

1 Finely slice the steak. Place it in a bowl, sprinkle in the cornflour, chilli flakes and seasoning, and toss well. Set aside.

2 Place the red cabbage and carrot in a bowl and mix well. Pour in the vinegar, stir well and set aside for 10–15 minutes. At the end of that time add the coriander and peanuts.

3 Heat a frying pan over a medium heat and add the coconut oil. When it is just starting to smoke, add the steak, ensuring the strips are separated. Cook for 1–2 minutes on each side, or until nice and crisp. Using a slotted spoon, transfer the strips to a plate lined with kitchen paper and pat dry.

4 Place the salad in a serving bowl and top with the crispy beef. Serve with the lime wedges.

**Prep: 10 minutes + 15 minutes marinating /
Cook: 4–5 minutes / Skill: simple**

SMOKED MACKEREL SALAD

SERVES 1

1 tbsp pumpkin seeds
½ small cucumber,
chopped into 1cm dice
small handful of dill,
finely chopped
2 smoked mackerel fillets
(about 75g each)

Energy (kCal) 565/serving	
Fat (g) 44	Fibre (g) 2
Sat fat (g) 8.5	Protein (g) 37.5
Carbs (g) 4	Salt (g) 2.8
Sugar (g) 2	

1 Preheat the grill until very hot.

2 Place the pumpkin seeds, cucumber and dill in a bowl. Stir well.

3 Place the mackerel in a baking tray, skin side up, and cook under the grill until the skin starts to blister. Chop each fillet into 5–6 pieces and add to the salad. Give it all a good toss and serve.

Prep: 10 minutes / Cook: 10 minutes / Skill: simple

SMOKED TROUT WITH CUCUMBER, CELERY & OLIVE SALAD

SERVES 1

¼ cucumber, chopped
    into 1cm dice
3 celery sticks, finely
    sliced at an angle
2 tbsp pitted green olives,
    roughly chopped
small handful of dill,
    roughly chopped
1 tbsp olive oil
2 x 75g smoked trout fillets
salt and pepper

Energy (kCal) 385/serving	
Fat (g) 26	Fibre (g) 3.5
Sat fat (g) 4	Protein (g) 34
Carbs (g) 2	Salt (g) 3
Sugar (g) 2	

1 Place the cucumber, celery, olives and dill in a bowl. Add the olive oil and salt and pepper. Toss well.

2 Transfer the salad to a serving bowl, top with the trout and serve.

Prep: 10 minutes / Skill: simple

THAI SALAD WITH TURKEY ESCALOPE

SERVES 1

1 tsp coconut oil
1 turkey escalope,
   about 175–225g
juice of ½ lime
salt and pepper

For the salad

¼ red onion, finely chopped
¼ red chilli, finely chopped
1 tsp fish sauce
1 pinch grated fresh ginger
6 mint leaves, finely chopped
50g roasted peanuts

Energy (kCal) 510/serving	
Fat (g) 28	Fibre (g) 0.5
Sat fat (g) 7.5	Protein (g) 58
Carbs (g) 8	Salt (g) 1.5
Sugar (g) 4.5	

1 Preheat the oven to 180°C/Fan 160°C/Gas 4.

2 First make the salad: place all the ingredients in a bowl and toss well. Set aside.

3 Heat a frying pan over a medium heat and add the coconut oil. Season the turkey with salt and pepper and fry for 1 minute on each side. Transfer the turkey to the oven for another 5–6 minutes, or until cooked through. Allow to cool slightly before slicing into 6–8 pieces.

4 Place the salad in a serving bowl and top with the turkey slices. Squeeze the lime juice over the meat and enjoy.

Prep: 15 minutes / Cook: 5–6 minutes / Skill: simple

ASIAN MANGO SALAD WITH ROAST CHICKEN

SERVES 1

1 skinless chicken breast
pinch of Chinese
　five-spice powder
salt and pepper

For the salad

flesh from ½ mango,
　sliced into 3–4 pieces
1 spring onion, finely sliced
small handful of coriander,
　roughly chopped
¼ red chilli, finely chopped
grated zest and juice of ½ lime
6 cherry tomatoes, halved
1 carrot, peeled and grated
1 tsp fish sauce
1 tsp dark soy sauce

Energy (kCal) 276/serving	
Fat (g) 3	Fibre (g) 7.5
Sat fat (g) 1	Protein (g) 38
Carbs (g) 21	Salt (g) 2.4
Sugar (g) 20	

1 Preheat the oven to 180°C/Fan 160°C/Gas 4.

2 Place the chicken breast in a roasting tray and season with the five-spice powder, salt and pepper. Roast for 10–12 minutes, or until cooked through. Allow to cool before cutting into 6 pieces.

3 Place the mango flesh in a large bowl. Add all the remaining salad ingredients and toss well.

4 Serve the salad in a bowl with the chicken slices arranged on top.

Prep: 15 minutes / Cook: 12 minutes / Skill: simple

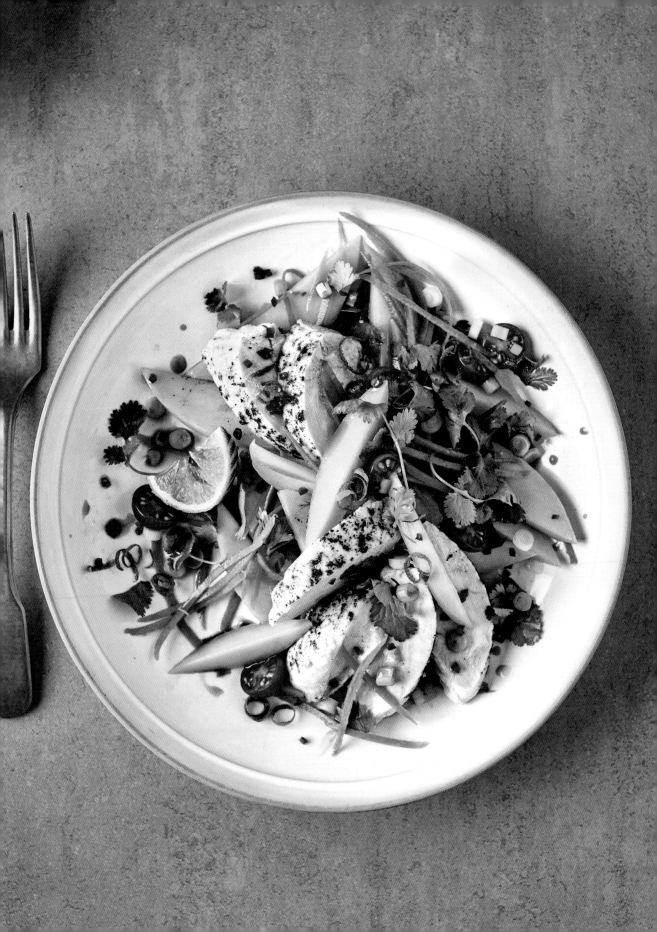

BEEF WITH FATTOUSH SALAD

SERVES 1

1 sirloin steak, about 175–225g
1 tbsp olive oil

For the salad
8 cherry tomatoes, halved
4 radishes, finely sliced
½ red onion, finely sliced
1 garlic clove, finely sliced
¼ cucumber, cut into chunks
½ red pepper, roughly diced
½ small handful of mint,
    roughly chopped
1 tbsp olive oil
salt and pepper

1 First make the salad: place all the ingredients in a bowl and mix well. Set aside.

2 Heat a frying pan over a high heat. Season the steak with salt and pepper and rub the olive oil into both sides of it. Place in the hot pan and cook for 2–3 minutes on each side. Allow the steak to rest for 5 minutes before slicing.

3 To serve, spoon the salad onto a serving plate and top with the sliced steak.

**Prep: 15 minutes + 5 minutes resting /
Cook: 6 minutes / Skill: simple**

Energy (kCal) 349/serving	
Fat (g) 11	Fibre (g) 6.5
Sat fat (g) 6	Protein (g) 20
Carbs (g) 39	Salt (g) 2.3
Sugar (g) 10	

PRAWN LETTUCE CUPS

SERVES 1

¼ red chilli, finely chopped
1 spring onion, finely chopped
small handful of coriander,
    finely chopped
100g cooked peeled prawns
2 tbsp cottage cheese
2 tsp curry powder
4 baby gem lettuce leaves

1 Put the chilli, spring onion and coriander in a bowl. Add the prawns. Toss to combine.

2 In a separate bowl, mix together the cottage cheese and curry powder.

3 Arrange the lettuce leaves on a plate. Spoon some cottage cheese into each leaf, then top with the prawn mixture and serve.

Prep: 10 minutes / Skill: simple

Energy (kCal) 137/serving	
Fat (g) 4	Fibre (g) 4
Sat fat (g) 1	Protein (g) 21
Carbs (g) 4.5	Salt (g) 1.9
Sugar (g) 2	

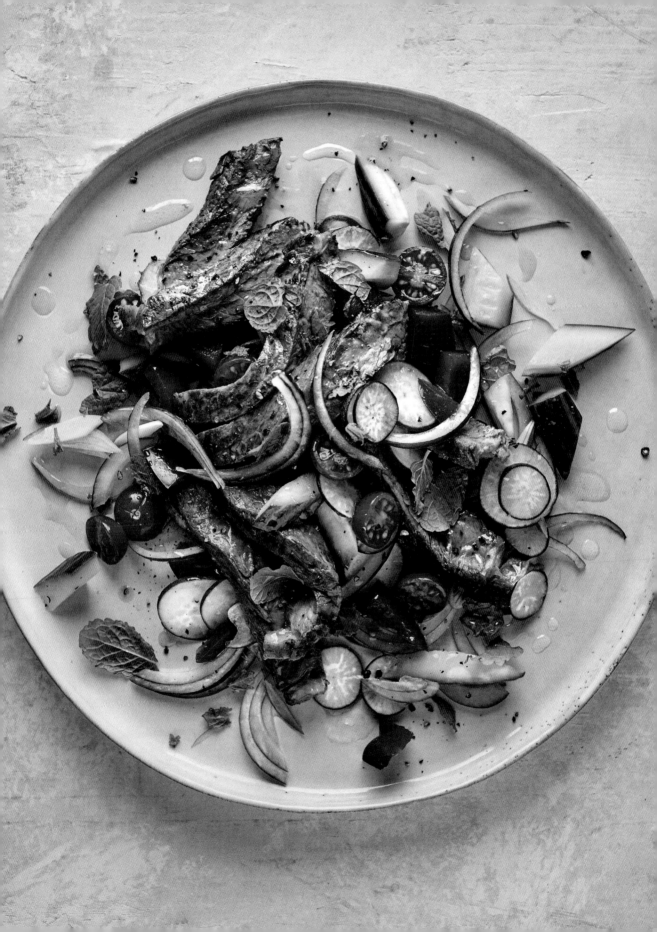

PORK MEATBALLS WITH BEETROOT & AVOCADO SALAD

SERVES 1

150g minced pork
1 tsp dried chilli flakes
1 tbsp freshly grated
    Parmesan cheese
salt and pepper

For the salad
3–4 small cooked beetroot,
    peeled and quartered
½ small orange, peeled
    and sliced into rounds
½ ripe avocado, sliced
1 tbsp pumpkin seeds, toasted

Energy (kCal) 647/serving	
Fat (g) 41	Fibre (g) 9
Sat fat (g) 12.5	Protein (g) 44
Carbs (g) 22	Salt (g) 0.85
Sugar (g) 18	

1 Place the pork in a bowl and add the chilli flakes, Parmesan and seasoning. Mix together gently, then divide into 6–8 equal pieces. Roll each one into a ball, place on a plate and put into the fridge for 30 minutes.

2 Preheat the oven to 180°C/Fan 160°C/Gas 4.

3 Place all the salad ingredients in a bowl and toss gently to combine.

4 Put the chilled meatballs in a roasting tray and place in the oven for 8–10 minutes, or until cooked through.

5 To serve, place the salad in a serving bowl and top with the meatballs.

**Prep: 10 minutes + 30 minutes chilling /
Cook: 8–10 minutes / Skill: simple**

ROASTED HAM WITH FETA, ROCKET & OMEGA SEEDS

SERVES 1

3 slices of good-quality
    dry-cured parma ham
6 cherry tomatoes, halved
large handful of rocket leaves
1 tbsp omega seeds
50g feta cheese

Energy (kCal) 284/serving	
Fat (g) 21	Fibre (g) 3
Sat fat (g) 9	Protein (g) 2
Carbs (g) 3	Salt (g) 2.1
Sugar (g) 3	

1 Preheat the oven to 200°C/Fan 180°C/Gas 6.

2 Spread the ham out in a roasting tray and place in the oven for 8–10 minutes, or until crisp. Set aside.

3 Add the tomatoes, rocket and omega seeds to a bowl, then crumble in the feta. Toss well, then transfer to a serving bowl. Tear the crispy ham over the salad and serve.

Prep: 10 minutes / Cook: 8–10 minutes / Skill: simple

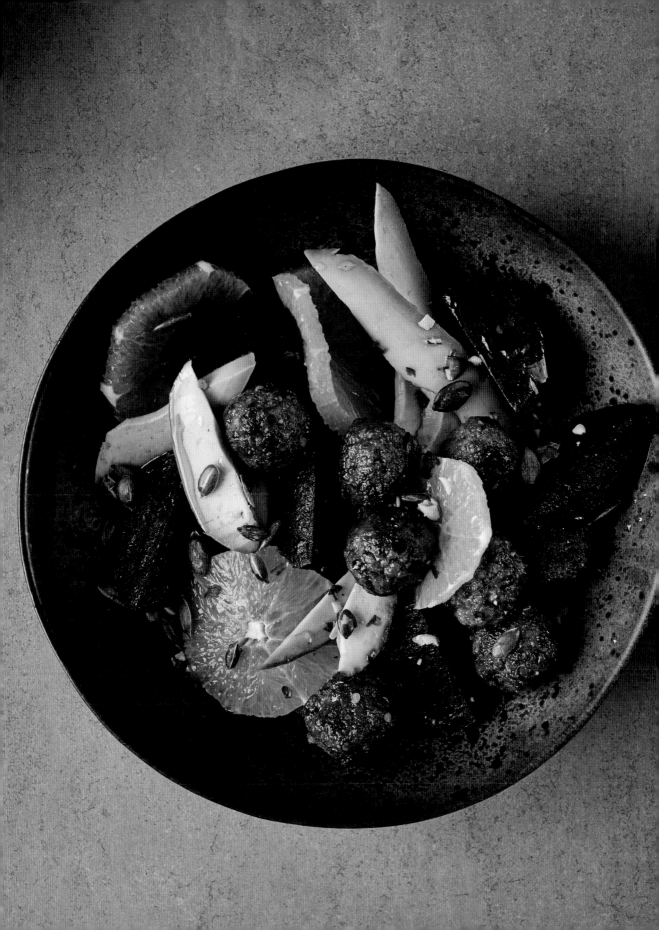

TURKEY KATSU CURRY WITH BROWN RICE

SERVES 1
2 tsp (10g) plain flour
20g panko breadcrumbs
1 small egg
1 turkey escalope, about 175g
1 tbsp coconut oil

For the sauce
2 garlic cloves
1 tbsp curry powder
2 tsp dark soy sauce
2 tbsp tomato ketchup
1 tbsp runny honey
pinch of ground ginger
1 tbsp peanut butter

For the rice
75g brown rice

Energy (kCal) 974/serving	
Fat (g) 29	Fibre (g) 7
Sat fat (g) 14	Protein (g) 65
Carbs (g) 108	Salt (g) 2.9
Sugar (g) 26	

1 Preheat the oven to 180°C/Fan 160°C/Gas 4.

2 Start by putting all the sauce ingredients in a saucepan. Place over a medium heat and bring to a gentle simmer: do not let it boil. Cook for 15–20 minutes, then transfer to a food processor and blend until smooth. Set aside.

3 Bring a small pan of salted water to the boil, add the rice and cook for 25–30 minutes, or until tender. Drain well, then stir in the teaspoonful of coconut oil and set aside.

4 Put the flour and breadcrumbs on separate plates. Break the egg into a shallow bowl and whisk well. Now dip the turkey first into the flour, then into the egg and finally into the breadcrumbs, making sure both sides are well coated.

5 Heat a frying pan over a medium heat and add the tablespoon of coconut oil. Fry the turkey for 2 minutes on each side, or until golden brown. Transfer to the oven for 6–7 minutes, or until cooked through.

6 To serve, place the rice in a bowl, top with the turkey and pour some of the sauce over it. Any remaining sauce can be stored in an airtight container and kept for up to 3 days.

Prep: 15 minutes / Cook: 50 minutes / Skill: simple

SPICED CHICKEN WITH MOLE SAUCE & SWEET POTATO

SERVES 1

1 sweet potato, unpeeled
1 skinless chicken breast
2–3 good pinches of
   Cajun spice
juice of 1 lime

For the sauce

2 red chillies,
   roughly chopped
2 plum tomatoes,
   roughly chopped
¼ Spanish onion,
   roughly chopped
2 garlic cloves
1 tbsp almonds
1 tsp raisins
1 tsp ground cumin
pinch of ground cinnamon
1 tsp cocoa powder
small handful of
   fresh coriander

Energy (kCal) 562/serving	
Fat (g) 13	Fibre (g) 13
Sat fat (g) 2	Protein (g) 46
Carbs (g) 60	Salt (g) 2.6
Sugar (g) 26	

1 Preheat the oven to 180°C/Fan 160°C/Gas 4.

2 Place the sweet potato in a roasting tray and bake for 25–30 minutes, or until soft to the touch.

3 Meanwhile, make the sauce. Place all the ingredients for it in a food processor and blend until smooth. Add 100ml water, blend briefly to combine, then pour into a saucepan and cook over a very low heat for 15 minutes.

4 Place the chicken breast in a bowl and season with the Cajun spice, making sure all sides are coated. Transfer to a roasting tray and roast for 12–15 minutes, or until cooked through.

5 Cut the sweet potato in half lengthways and squeeze the lime juice over the flesh. Place in a shallow serving bowl and put the chicken beside it. Pour the mole sauce over the chicken and serve.

Prep: 15 minutes / Cook: 45 minutes / Skill: simple

SEARED TUNA WITH LEMON POTATO SALAD & SALSA VERDE

SERVES 1

1 tuna steak, about 150g
1 tsp olive oil
juice of ½ lemon

For the potato salad

1 large potato, peeled and diced
1 tsp finely chopped chives
2 tsp olive oil
grated zest and juice
    of ½ lemon

For the salsa

1 garlic clove
1 tbsp capers
handful of baby spinach leaves
small handful of basil leaves
3–4 tbsp olive oil
1 tbsp white wine vinegar
salt and pepper

Energy (kCal) 765/serving	
Fat (g) 43	Fibre (g) 5
Sat fat (g) 6.5	Protein (g) 43
Carbs (g) 47	Salt (g) 0.3
Sugar (g) 2	

1 First make the salad. Place the potato in a saucepan, cover with water and bring to the boil. Cook for 10–15 minutes, or until tender. Drain well and place in a bowl. Add the chives, oil, lemon zest and juice. Toss well, then set aside.

2 Place all the salsa ingredients in a food processor and pulse until you have a chunky mixture. Season with salt and pepper.

3 Heat a griddle pan over a high heat. Season the tuna with salt and pepper and rub the olive oil into both sides of it. Cook on the griddle for 1½–2 minutes on each side, then squeeze the lemon juice over it.

4 To serve, place the potato salad in a bowl and top with the tuna steak. Pour the salsa verde over it and serve.

Prep: 10 minutes / Cook: 20–25 minutes / Skill: simple

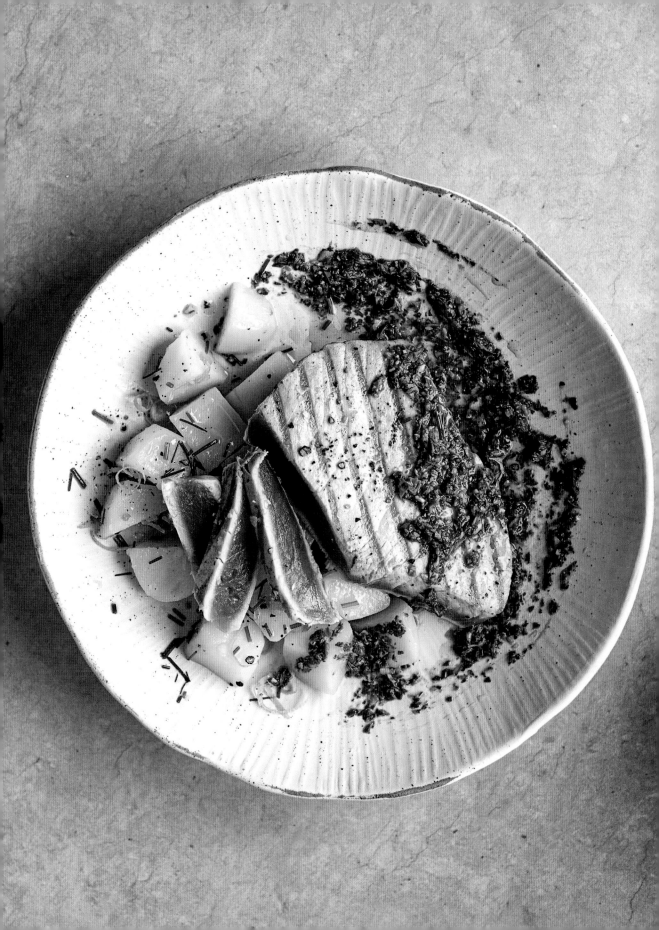

PORK FILLET WITH WHITE BEAN & CHORIZO STEW

SERVES 1

1 x 175–225g slice of pork fillet
1 tbsp olive oil
juice of ½ lemon

For the stew

1 x 400g tin chopped tomatoes
200g cooked butterbeans
50g piece of chorizo,
    roughly chopped
2 garlic cloves
1 tbsp olive oil
handful of baby spinach leaves
salt and pepper

Energy (kCal) 883/serving	
Fat (g) 46	Fibre (g) 16
Sat fat (g) 12	Protein (g) 67
Carbs (g) 40	Salt (g) 2
Sugar (g) 17	

1 Preheat the oven to 180°C/Fan 160°C/Gas 4.

2 To make the stew, put the tomatoes, butterbeans, chorizo and garlic in a saucepan, add the olive oil and season with salt and pepper. Place over a medium heat, bring to a bubble, then simmer for 15–20 minutes. Stir in the spinach, check the seasoning and set aside.

3 Meanwhile, season the pork with salt and pepper and rub the olive oil all over it. Heat a frying pan over a high heat. Add the pork and cook until browned all over. Transfer to the oven for another 10–12 minutes, or until cooked through. Allow to rest for 5 minutes before slicing into 5–6 pieces.

4 To serve, pour the bean stew into a serving bowl. Squeeze the lemon juice over the pork, then place it on top of the stew.

Prep: 10 minutes / Cook: 32 minutes + 5 minutes resting / Skill: simple

HARISSA-GRILLED SARDINES WITH WALNUT POTATO SALAD

SERVES 1

4–5 fresh sardines,
  gutted and scaled
1 tbsp harissa paste
juice of 1 lemon
salt and pepper

For the salad

1 potato, peeled and diced
1 tbsp olive oil
small handful of coriander,
  finely chopped
1 tbsp walnut halves,
  roughly chopped
seeds from ½ pomegranate

Energy (kCal) 692/serving	
Fat (g) 35	Fibre (g) 7
Sat fat (g) 6	Protein (g) 47
Carbs (g) 44	Salt (g) 0.9
Sugar (g) 9	

1 Place the sardines in a shallow bowl. Season with salt and pepper, then rub all over with the harissa. Place in the fridge for 30 minutes.

2 Preheat the grill until very hot.

3 Meanwhile, make the salad. Place the potato in a saucepan of salted water and bring to the boil. Cook for 15 minutes, or until tender. Drain, then transfer to a bowl. Add the remaining ingredients plus salt and pepper, mix well, then set aside.

4 Place the sardines on a grill a tray and grill for 3–4 minutes on each side.

5 To serve, place the potato salad on a serving plate and top with the sardines. Squeeze over the lemon juice and serve.

Prep: 15 minutes + 30 minutes marinating / Cook: 20–25 minutes / Skill: simple

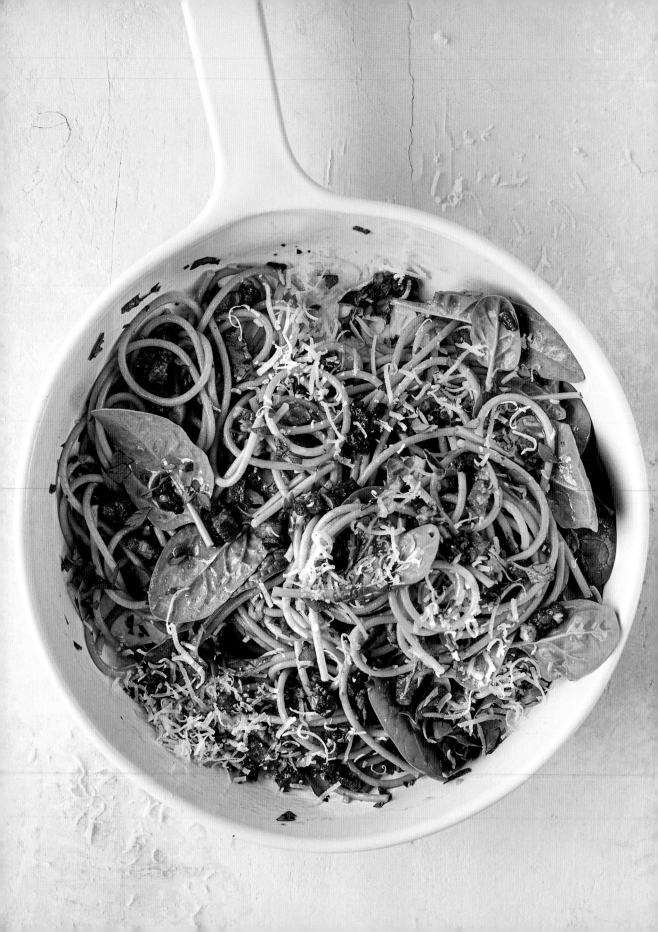

SPAGHETTI & PANCETTA, CHILLI, PARSLEY AND PARMESAN

SERVES 1

75g wholewheat spaghetti
knob of butter
50g pancetta cubes
½ red chilli, finely chopped
1 garlic clove, finely chopped
handful of baby spinach leaves
2 tbsp parsley leaves,
    roughly choped
1 tbsp freshly grated
    Parmesan cheese
1 tbsp olive oil
salt and pepper

Energy (kCal) 646/serving	
Fat (g) 37	Fibre (g) 16
Sat fat (g) 13	Protein (g) 25
Carbs (g) 50	Salt (g) 2.3
Sugar (g) 3	

1 Bring a saucepan of lightly salted water to the boil and cook the pasta for 8 minutes, or until tender. Drain well.

2 Meanwhile, heat a large sauté pan over a high heat, add the butter and fry the pancetta until crisp and golden brown. Add the chilli and garlic and continue cooking for 2–3 minutes.

3 Toss the cooked spaghetti into the pancetta mixture, along with the spinach, parsley, Parmesan and olive oil. Toss well. Check the seasoning and serve in a large pasta bowl.

Prep: 10 minutes / **Cook: 15 minutes** / **Skill: simple**

FILLET OF COD WITH ROASTED SQUASH POLENTA

SERVES 1

1 cod fillet, about 200–225g
juice of ½ lemon

For the polenta

¼ butternut squash, peeled and
    cut into 6 wedges
1 tbsp olive oil
1 tsp dried chilli flakes
200ml semi-skimmed milk
50g fine polenta (cornmeal)
2–3 tbsp freshly grated
    Parmesan cheese
salt and pepper

Energy (kCal) 850/serving	
Fat (g) 37	Fibre (g) 8
Sat fat (g) 11	Protein (g) 56
Carbs (g) 68	Salt (g) 1.1
Sugar (g) 22	

1 Preheat the oven to 180°C/Fan 160°C/Gas 4.

2 Place the squash in a baking tray and sprinkle with the olive oil and chilli flakes. Season with salt and pepper and roast for 10–15 minutes, or until tender. Set aside.

3 Pour the milk into a large saucepan, bring to the boil, then reduce the heat to a gentle simmer. Pour in the polenta, stirring continuously, and cook for 10 minutes. You might need to add a little extra milk or water if the polenta becomes too stiff; it should be the consistency of mashed potato. Season with salt and pepper, then fold in the roasted squash and the Parmesan. Do not mash. Remove from the heat, cover and set aside.

4 Place the cod in a roasting tray, season with salt and pepper and roast for 8–10 minutes, or until cooked through.

5 To serve, spoon the polenta into a serving bowl, top with the roasted cod and squeeze over the lemon juice.

Prep: 15 minutes / Cook: 35 minutes / Skill: moderate

CHICKEN, COCONUT, CHICKPEA & SPINACH CURRY WITH PILAU RICE

SERVES 1

2 tsp coconut oil
½ onion, finely sliced
1 garlic clove, finely sliced
pinch of ground cumin
2 tsp curry powder
1 cardamom pod
1 skinless chicken breast
1 x 200ml tin low-fat coconut
　milk, well shaken
200ml chicken stock
50g cooked chickpeas
2 handfuls of baby
　spinach leaves
salt and pepper

For the rice

2 cardamom pods
pinch of ground cinnamon
2 cloves
75g brown rice
1 tbsp sultanas

Energy (kCal) 824/serving	
Fat (g) 28	Fibre (g) 11
Sat fat (g) 19	Protein (g) 51
Carbs (g) 85	Salt (g) 0.4
Sugar (g) 17	

1 Heat a large saucepan over a medium heat, add the tablespoon of coconut oil and fry the onion and garlic for 2–3 minutes. Stir in the cumin, curry powder and cardamom and continue cooking for 2 minutes.

2 Slice the chicken breast into 4–5 pieces and add to the saucepan. Cook for 2 minutes, then add the coconut milk and stock. Turn the heat down and simmer gently for 15–20 minutes.

3 Meanwhile, to make the rice, heat another saucepan over a high heat and add the cardamom, cinnamon and cloves and cook for 1 minute, taking care that nothing burns. Stir in the rice. Cover with water and bring to the boil, then cook for 10 minutes, or until tender. Drain well and stir in the sultanas. Check the seasoning.

4 About 2 minutes before the chicken is ready, add the chickpeas and spinach to heat through. Check the seasoning.

5 To serve, spoon the rice into a bowl and top with the chicken curry.

Prep: 15 minutes / **Cook: 50 minutes** / **Skill: simple**

MINI CHICKEN PASTILLA

SERVES 2

3 sheets filo or brik pastry
1–2 tbsp melted butter

For the filling

1 skinless chicken breast
1 tsp butter
½ onion, finely chopped
pinch of saffron strands
pinch of ground cinnamon
pinch of ground cumin
50g flaked almonds
2 eggs
small handful of parsley,
   finely chopped
6 mint leaves, finely chopped
salt and pepper

Energy (kCal) 1114/serving	
Fat (g) 60	Fibre (g) 1.5
Sat fat (g) 16.5	Protein (g) 74
Carbs (g) 68	Salt (g) 1.7
Sugar (g) 8	

1 Preheat the oven to 200°C/Fan 180°C/Gas 6.

2 First make the filling. Season the chicken breast with salt and pepper, then chop it into 5–6 pieces. Heat a large saucepan over a medium heat and melt the butter in it. Add the chicken and cook for 4–5 minutes, or until browned. Add the onion and cook for 2–3 minutes. Once it is slightly translucent, add the spices and almonds and cook for a further 4–5 minutes. Finally, add 150ml water and cook for 10–15 minutes.

3 Once the water has reduced, remove just the chicken from the pan and set aside on a plate. Crack the eggs into the onion mixture and stir until they have scrambled.

4 Return the chicken to the pan, add the parsley and mint and stir well. Taste and adjust the seasoning.

5 Brush a sheet of the pastry with melted butter, lay another sheet on top and brush again with butter. Place the remaining sheet on top. Now use this pastry 'sandwich' to line a 20–25cm ovenproof sauté pan or cake tin, leaving plenty overhanging the edge. Spoon the filling into the pastry case, then fold the overhanging pastry over the top to act as a lid. Brush generously with the remaining melted butter and bake for 15 minutes, or until brown and crisp.

6 Allow the pastilla to cool slightly before removing it from the pan or tin and serving.

Prep: 20 minutes / Cook: 35–40 minutes / Skill: moderate

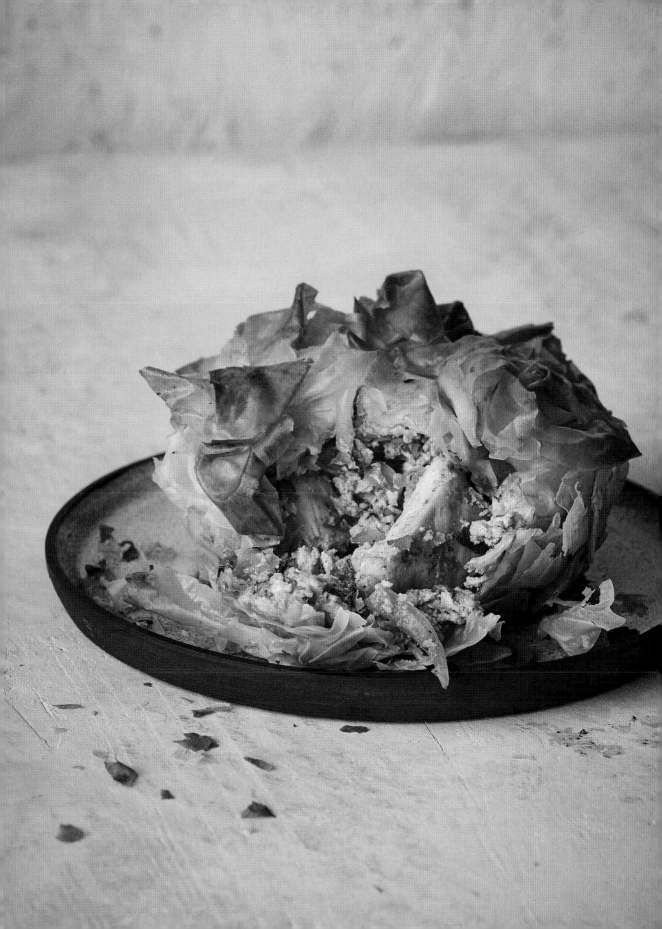

CURRIED LAMB CUTLETS WITH YOGHURT & SPICED BULGUR WHEAT

SERVES 1

4 lamb cutlets
1 tbsp curry powder
2 tbsp natural yoghurt

For the spiced bulgur

75g bulgur wheat
2 tsp curry powder
small handful of coriander,
    finely chopped
1 tbsp raisins
1 tbsp pumpkin seeds
1 tbsp whole almonds,
    roughly chopped
salt and pepper

Energy (kCal) 910/serving	
Fat (g) 36	Fibre (g) 14
Sat fat (g) 9	Protein (g) 61
Carbs (g) 77	Salt (g) 0.7
Sugar (g) 14	

1 Put the lamb cutlets in a bowl along with the curry powder and yoghurt and mix well. Place in the fridge for 30 minutes.

2 Put the bulgur wheat and curry powder in a small saucepan, cover with water and bring to the boil. Cook over a high heat for 15–20 minutes, or until tender. Drain well, then transfer to a bowl. Add the coriander, raisins, pumpkin seeds and almonds. Season with salt and pepper and stir to combine.

3 Heat a griddle pan over a high heat. When smoking hot, add the lamb cutlets and cook for 3–4 minutes on each side. (This will make them medium rare, so cook a little longer if you want no trace of pink.)

4 To serve, place the bulgur mixture on a serving plate and top with the lamb cutlets.

**Prep: 15 minutes + 30 minutes marinating /
Cook: 30 minutes / Skill: simple**

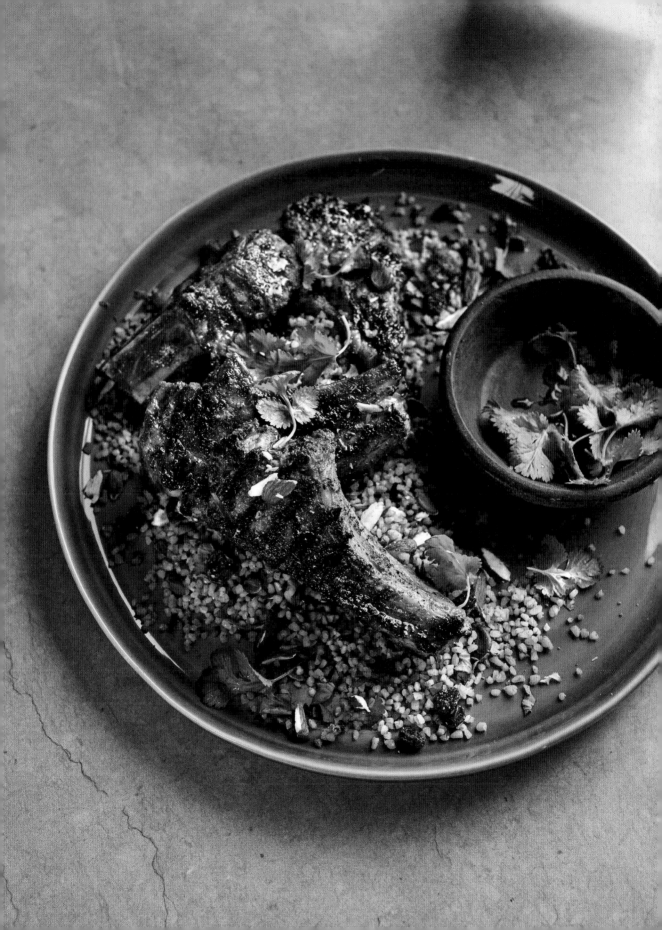

FILLET OF BEEF WITH SPINACH YOGHURT SAUCE & ROCKET SALAD

SERVES 1

1 x 200g fillet steak
2 tsp olive oil

For the spinach yoghurt

1 garlic clove, roughly chopped
¼ red chilli, roughly chopped
2 tbsp Greek yoghurt
large handful of baby
   spinach leaves
salt and pepper

For the salad

5–6 cherry tomatoes, halved
1 tbsp freshly grated
   Parmesan cheese
handful of rocket leaves

Energy (kCal) 457/serving	
Fat (g) 26	Fibre (g) 1.5
Sat fat (g) 11.5	Protein (g) 51
Carbs (g) 3	Salt (g) 0.6
Sugar (g) 3	

1 First make the spinach yoghurt. Place the garlic and chilli in a food processor along with the yoghurt and spinach and blend until smooth. Season with salt and pepper and set aside.

2 Heat a frying pan over a medium heat. Season the steak with salt and pepper and rub the olive oil all over it. Place in the hot pan and cook for 3–4 minutes on each side, or until caramelised. Remove from the pan and allow to rest for 5 minutes.

3 To make the salad, place the tomatoes in a bowl with the Parmesan and rocket. Toss to combine.

4 Slice the steak and arrange on a plate. Spoon over the sauce and serve with the salad.

Prep: 10 minutes / Cook: 8 minutes + 5 minutes resting / Skill: simple

SESAME-CRUSTED TUNA STEAK WITH TOMATO & SOY SALAD

SERVES 1

1–2 tbsp sesame seeds
1 x 150g tuna steak
2 plum tomatoes, quartered
5 basil leaves, finely sliced
2 spring onions, finely sliced
1 tbsp dark soy sauce
2 tsp rice wine vinegar
olive oil, for griddling

Energy (kCal) 390/serving	
Fat (g) 21	Fibre (g) 4.5
Sat fat (g) 3.5	Protein (g) 37
Carbs (g) 11.5	Salt (g) 2.3
Sugar (g) 11	

1 Sprinkle the sesame seeds onto a plate. Dip the tuna steak in them to coat evenly on both sides.

2 Combine the tomatoes, basil and spring onions in a bowl. Pour over the soy sauce and vinegar and toss well.

3 Heat a griddle pan on a high heat. Drizzle the olive oil into the pan and add the tuna. Cook for 1–2 minutes on each side, or until the sesame seeds are nicely coloured.

4 To serve, place the tomato salad on a plate and serve the tuna alongside.

Prep: 10 minutes / Cook: 5 minutes / Skill: simple

ROASTED SALMON WITH PEAS & ASPARAGUS

SERVES 1

1 x 150g salmon fillet
75g fresh or frozen peas
6 asparagus spears
1 garlic clove, finely chopped
2 tbsp parsley leaves,
    finely chopped
knob of butter
juice of ½ lemon
salt and pepper

Energy (kCal) 400/serving	
Fat (g) 25	Fibre (g) 7
Sat fat (g) 8.5	Protein (g) 9
Carbs (g) 10.5	Salt (g) 0.3
Sugar (g) 4	

1 Preheat the oven to 180°C/Fan 160°C/Gas 4.

2 Place the salmon in a roasting tray and season with salt and pepper. Roast for 8 minutes, or until cooked through.

3 Meanwhile, bring a small pan of lightly salted water to the boil. Throw in the peas and asparagus and cook for 60 seconds. Drain, then transfer to a bowl. Add the garlic and parsley, then season with salt and pepper. Stir in the butter until it has melted.

4 Tip the pea mixture into a bowl and top with the salmon. Squeeze over the lemon juice and serve.

Prep: 10 minutes / Cook: 8–10 minutes / Skill: simple

PORK, BEEF & ROSEMARY KEBABS WITH ROASTED VEGETABLE SALAD

SERVES 1

100g lean minced pork
100g lean minced beef
1 garlic clove, finely chopped
leaves from 1 sprig of
   rosemary, finely chopped
1 tbsp freshly grated
   Parmesan cheese
salt and pepper

For the salad

1 red pepper, deseeded and
   chopped into large chunks
½ aubergine, chopped into
   bite-sized pieces
1 tbsp olive oil
8 cherry tomatoes, halved
¼ red onion, finely sliced
1 tbsp dill leaves, finely
   chopped

Energy (kCal) 635/serving	
Fat (g) 35	Fibre (g) 10.5
Sat fat (g) 13	Protein (g) 54
Carbs (g) 18	Salt (g) 0.9
Sugar (g) 17	

1 Preheat the oven to 180°C/Fan 160°C/Gas 4.

2 Using a spoon, mix the minced pork and beef together in a bowl. Add the garlic, rosemary, Parmesan and seasoning and mix again. Divide the mixture into 8 equal pieces, then roll each one into a ball. Transfer to a plate and place in the fridge for 30 minutes.

3 Meanwhile, to make the salad, place the red pepper and aubergine in a roasting tray. Season with salt and pepper and drizzle over the olive oil. Roast for 20 minutes, or until the vegetables are tender.

4 Place the tomatoes and onion in a large bowl. Once the roasted vegetables are ready, add them to the tomatoes along with the dill and mix well.

5 Thread the chilled meatballs onto 2 skewers. (If using wooden skewers, make sure you soak them in water for 30 minutes before use so they won't catch fire.) Put the kebabs in a roasting tray and place in the oven for 10–12 minutes, or until cooked through.

6 To serve, place the roasted vegetable salad on a plate and top with the meatball kebabs.

**Prep: 15 minutes + 30 minutes chilling /
Cook: 35 minutes / Skill: simple**

CHICKEN KEBABS MARINATED WITH CHILLI & HONEY

SERVES 1

2 skinless chicken breasts
1 garlic clove
½ red chilli
1 tbsp runny honey
1 tsp ground cumin
juice of 1 lemon
2 tbsp coriander leaves
salt and pepper

Energy (kCal) 376/serving	
Fat (g) 4	Fibre (g) 3
Sat fat (g) 1	Protein (g) 74
Carbs (g) 14.5	Salt (g) 0.5
Sugar (g) 14.5	

1 Cut each chicken breast into 4 strips and place in a large bowl.

2 Place all the remaining ingredients in a food processor and blend until smooth. Pour the mixture over the chicken and leave to marinate for at least 30 minutes, but longer if you can.

3 Thread the chicken pieces onto 2 skewers. (If using wooden skewers, make sure you soak them in water for 30 minutes before use so they won't catch fire.)

4 Heat a griddle pan over a high heat and cook the kebabs for 5–6 minutes on each side, or until cooked through. Serve straight away.

Prep: 10 minutes + 30 minutes marinating / Cook: 10–12 minutes / Skill: simple

CHICKEN & OLIVE STEW

SERVES 1

1 tbsp olive oil
1 garlic clove
½ onion
sprig of thyme
1 skinless chicken breast
1 x 400g tin chopped tomatoes
50g pitted green olives
1 tbsp capers
2 tbsp parsley leaves
grated zest and juice
    of ½ lemon
salt and pepper

Energy (kCal) 431/serving	
Fat (g) 19	Fibre (g) 7
Sat fat (g) 3	Protein (g) 42
Carbs (g) 21	Salt (g) 1.9
Sugar (g) 19	

1 Preheat the oven to 180°C/Fan 160°C/Gas 4.

2 Heat the oil in a flameproof casserole dish or sauté pan over a medium heat. Add the garlic and onion and fry for 2–3 minutes. Stir in the thyme.

3 Season the chicken with salt and pepper, add to the pan and brown on all sides.

4 Stir in the tomatoes, olives and capers, then lower the heat, cover the dish or pan and transfer to the oven. Cook for 20–25 minutes, or until the chicken is cooked through and the sauce has reduced slightly.

5 Stir the parsley into the stew. Add the lemon zest and juice, stir again and serve.

Prep: 15 minutes / Cook: 25–30 minutes / Skill: simple

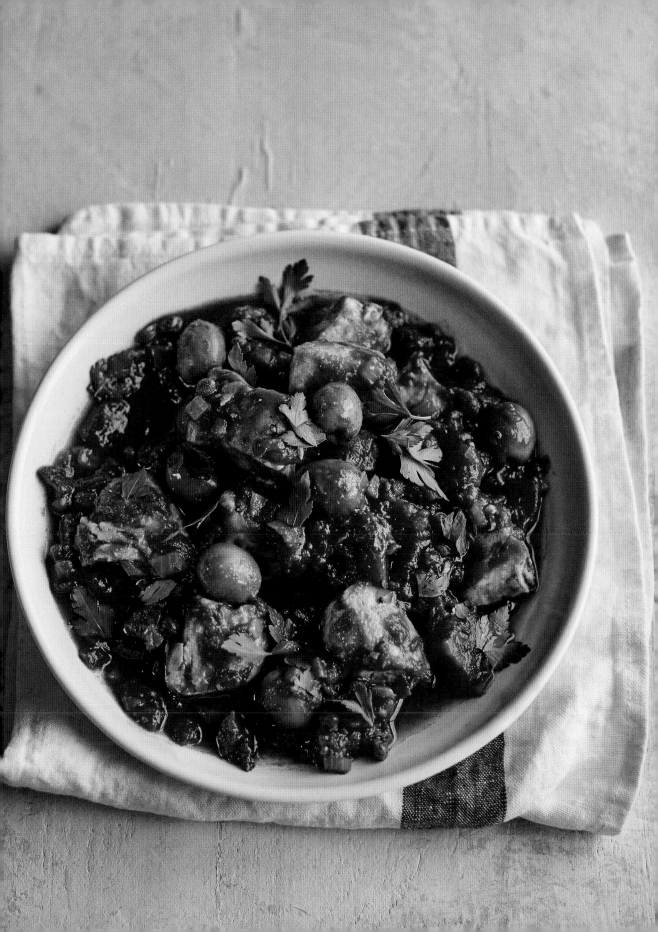

LAMB IN YOGHURT WITH CARROT SALAD

SERVES 1

200g lean minced lamb
1 garlic clove, finely chopped
2 tbsp coriander leaves,
    finely chopped
1 tsp ground cumin
pinch of ground cinnamon
50g fresh or defrosted
    frozen peas
2 tbsp Greek yoghurt
salt and pepper

For the salad

2 carrots, peeled and grated
¼ red onion, finely chopped
2 tbsp finely chopped dill

Energy (kCal) 581/serving	
Fat (g) 32	Fibre (g) 11
Sat fat (g) 15	Protein (g) 45
Carbs (g) 23	Salt (g) 0.7
Sugar (g) 17	

1 Place the lamb in a large bowl. Add the garlic and coriander and mix well. Sprinkle in the cumin, cinnamon and peas and mix again. Season with salt and pepper. Divide the mixture into 8 equal pieces and roll each one into a ball. Transfer to a plate and place in the fridge for 30 minutes.

2 Preheat the oven to 180°C/Fan 160°C/Gas 4.

3 Meanwhile, make the salad. Put the carrots and red onion in a bowl. Add the dill and mix well.

4 Place the chilled meatballs in a roasting tray and roast for 10 minutes, or until cooked through. Transfer to a bowl, pour in the yoghurt and gently stir together.

5 Place the carrot salad in a serving bowl, top with the meatballs and yoghurt and serve.

**Prep: 15 minutes + 30 minutes chilling /
Cook: 10–15 minutes / Skill: simple**

ROAST COD WITH ROASTED RED PEPPERS & PEPPER SAUCE

SERVES 1

2 red peppers
2 tbsp olive oil
1 garlic clove, finely chopped
½ onion, finely chopped
50ml vegetable stock
½ tsp sugar
1 x 400g tin chopped tomatoes
1 cod fillet, about 200–225g
juice of ½ lemon
salt and pepper

Energy (kCal) 534/serving	
Fat (g) 24	Fibre (g) 11
Sat fat (g) 3.5	Protein (g) 38
Carbs (g) 35	Salt (g) 0.8
Sugar (g) 33	

1 Preheat the oven to 200°C/Fan 180°C/Gas 6.

2 Put the peppers in a roasting tray and drizzle half the olive oil over them. Place in the oven for 10–20 minutes, or until soft and browned. Set aside until cool enough to handle, then remove the stalks. Finely slice one pepper and roughly chop the other one, keeping them separate.

3 Place a small saucepan over a medium heat and add the remaining olive oil. Fry the garlic and onion in it for 2–3 minutes. Add the roughly chopped pepper, the stock, sugar and tomatoes and simmer for 10–15 minutes. Check the seasoning, then blend in a food processor until smooth.

4 Place the cod in a roasting tray, season with salt and pepper and roast for 8 minutes, or until cooked through. When done, squeeze the lemon juice over it.

5 To serve, place the cod on a plate, pour the sauce over it and top with the finely sliced pepper.

Prep: 15 minutes / Cook: 40–45 minutes / Skill: simple

ROASTED PORK CHOP WITH ORANGE & FENNEL SALAD

SERVES 1

1 pork chop, on the bone
1 tbsp olive oil
salt and pepper

For the salad
½ fennel bulb, finely sliced
¼ red onion, finely sliced
1 tbsp white wine vinegar
1 tsp sugar
½ orange, peeled
   and segmented
2 tbsp dill leaves
2 tbsp pitted black olives,
   roughly chopped
salt and pepper

Energy (kCal) 433/serving	
Fat (g) 24	Fibre (g) 7.5
Sat fat (g) 4.5	Protein (g) 36
Carbs (g) 14	Salt (g) 0.1
Sugar (g) 13	

1 Preheat the oven to 200°C/Fan 180°C/Gas 6.

2 First make the salad. Place the fennel and onion in a large bowl. Add the vinegar and sugar, stir well and set aside for 10 minutes.

3 Add the orange, dill and olives and toss together. Set aside.

4 Heat an ovenproof frying pan over a high heat. Season the chop with salt and pepper, then rub the olive oil into both sides of it. Fry in the hot pan for 2–3 minutes on each side, or until golden brown. Transfer to the oven and cook for a further 5–6 minutes, or until cooked through. Allow to rest for 5 minutes.

5 To serve, spoon the salad onto a serving plate and top with the chop. Drizzle with any remaining pan juices.

Prep: 10 minutes / Cook: 12–15 minutes / Skill: simple

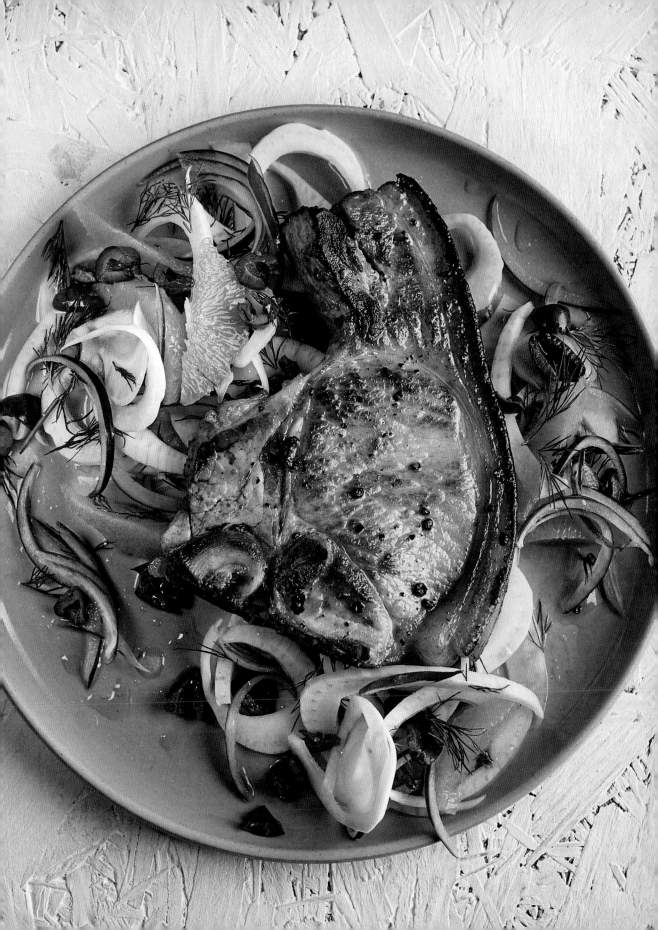

SMOOTHIES PRE-WORKOUT

All the following smoothie recipes serve one and take about two minutes to make. In each case, prepare all the ingredients as directed, then whizz in a blender. Pour into a glass and enjoy.

BLUEBERRY & AVOCADO SMOOTHIE

½ ripe avocado
2 tbsp Greek yoghurt
2 tsp runny honey
100g blueberries
1 tbsp peanut butter
100ml semi-skimmed milk

Energy (kCal) 461/serving	
Fat (g) 30	Fibre (g) 6
Sat fat (g) 10	Protein (g) 13
Carbs (g) 31	Salt (g) 0.4
Sugar (g) 28	

COCOA & OAT SMOOTHIE

200ml semi-skimmed milk
1 tbsp Greek yoghurt
25g porridge oats
½ tbsp flaxseed or linseed
1 tsp cocoa powder
½ ripe banana
½ scoop chocolate protein powder

Energy (kCal) 350/serving	
Fat (g) 11	Fibre (g) 5
Sat fat (g) 5	Protein (g) 23
Carbs (g) 37	Salt (g) 0.2
Sugar (g) 19	

GRAPEFRUIT, STRAWBERRY & PINEAPPLE SMOOTHIE

1 pink grapefruit, peeled and roughly chopped
¼ pineapple, peeled and roughly chopped
50g strawberries
2 tbsp Greek yoghurt
150ml water

Energy (kCal) 247/serving	
Fat (g) 4	Fibre (g) 9.5
Sat fat (g) 2	Protein (g) 4.5
Carbs (g) 43	Salt (g) trace
Sugar (g) 43	

KIWI & KALE SMOOTHIE

400ml semi-skimmed milk
handful of kale leaves
1 kiwi fruit, peeled
1 tbsp peanut butter
1 tsp runny honey
1 scoop vanilla protein powder

Energy (kCal) 429/serving	
Fat (g) 16	Fibre (g) 3.5
Sat fat (g) 7	Protein (g) 36.5
Carbs (g) 33	Salt (g) 0.7
Sugar (g) 32	

BANANA & WALNUT SMOOTHIE

500ml semi-skimmed milk
1 ripe banana
1 tbsp runny honey
8–10 walnut halves
1 scoop vanilla protein powder

Energy (kCal) 457/serving	
Fat (g) 9	Fibre (g) 1.5
Sat fat (g) 6	Protein (g) 35
Carbs (g) 57	Salt (g) 0.6
Sugar (g) 55	

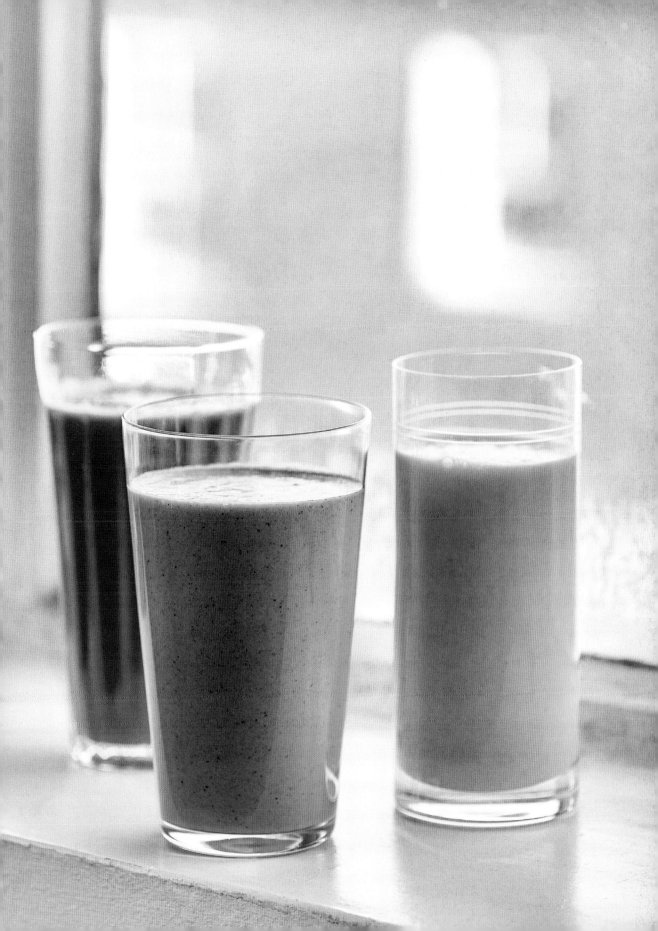

SMOOTHIES POST-WORKOUT

PEAR & GINGER SMOOTHIE

1 ripe pear, cored and roughly chopped
100ml coconut water
1cm piece fresh root ginger
1 tbsp Greek yoghurt
2 tsp runny honey
1 scoop vanilla protein powder

Energy (kCal) 216/serving	
Fat (g) 4	Fibre (g) 7
Sat fat (g) 2.5	Protein (g) 35
Carbs (g) 38	Salt (g) 0.3
Sugar (g) 38	

MANGO & TURMERIC SMOOTHIE

1 mango, peeled and stoned
½ tsp ground turmeric
1 tsp runny honey
100ml coconut water
2 tbsp Greek yoghurt

Energy (kCal) 216/serving	
Fat (g) 4	Fibre (g) 7
Sat fat (g) 2.5	Protein (g) 3.5
Carbs (g) 38	Salt (g) 0.3
Sugar (g) 38	

CHERRY & CHIA SMOOTHIE

100g fresh or frozen cherries, pitted
2 tsp runny honey
½ tsp ground turmeric
1 tsp chia seeds
2 tbsp Greek yoghurt
400ml semi-skimmed milk
1 scoop strawberry protein powder

Energy (kCal) 434/serving	
Fat (g) 12	Fibre (g) 3
Sat fat (g) 7	Protein (g) 34
Carbs (g) 45	Salt (g) 0.6
Sugar (g) 42	

HONEY & SESAME WAFERS

MAKES 12
50g butter
50g runny honey
25g light brown sugar
1 egg
1 tsp vanilla extract
75g wholemeal flour
¼ tsp baking powder
¼ tsp table salt
pinch of ground cinnamon
125g sesame seeds

Energy (kCal) 146/serving	
Fat (g) 10	Fibre (g) 2
Sat fat (g) 3.5	Protein (g) 4
Carbs (g) 9	Salt (g) 0.2
Sugar (g) 5	

1 Preheat the oven to 180°C/Fan 160°C/Gas 4. Line a baking sheet with baking parchment.

2 Put the butter, honey and sugar into a mixer and beat until light and fluffy. Add the egg and vanilla and beat again.

3 In a separate bowl combine the flour, baking powder, salt and cinnamon. Pour in the egg mixture, add the sesame seeds and mix well.

4 Place 12 teaspoonfuls of the mixture on the prepared sheet, ensuring they are evenly spaced.

5 Bake for 7–8 minutes, or until golden brown. Allow to cool before serving or storing in an airtight container.

Prep: 15 minutes / Cook: 7–8 minutes / Skill: simple

CHICKPEA & CHOCOLATE COOKIES

MAKES 8

1 x 400g tin chickpeas, drained
125g peanut butter
2 tbsp runny honey
pinch of salt
¼ tsp baking powder
¼ tsp bicarbonate of soda
200g chocolate chips

Energy (kCal) 277/serving	
Fat (g) 16	Fibre (g) 4
Sat fat (g) 7	Protein (g) 8
Carbs (g) 23	Salt (g) 0.3
Sugar (g) 18	

1 Preheat the oven to 180°C/Fan 160°C/Gas 4. Line a baking sheet with baking parchment.

2 Put all the ingredients, except the chocolate chips, into a food processor and blend until the mixture looks like cookie dough. Transfer to a large bowl and mix in the chocolate chips.

3 Using a tablespoon, place spoonfuls of the mixture on the prepared sheet, spacing them out evenly.

4 Bake for 20 minutes. Allow to cool before serving.

Prep: 10 minutes / Cook: 20 minutes / Skill: simple

ROASTED SALT & CHILLI ALMONDS

SERVES 1

150g unskinned almonds
1 tbsp coconut oil
1 tsp sea salt
½ tsp chilli flakes
1 tsp smoked paprika

Energy (kCal) 174/serving	
Fat (g) 16	Fibre (g) 0.5
Sat fat (g) 3	Protein (g) 6.5
Carbs (g) 1.5	Salt (g) 0.83
Sugar (g) 1	

1 Preheat the oven to 180°C/Fan 160°C/Gas 4.

2 Spread the almonds in a roasting tray and place in the oven for 10 minutes.

3 Transfer the hot nuts to a bowl, add all the remaining ingredients and stir well. Allow to cool before serving or storing in an airtight container.

Prep: 10 minutes / Cook: 10 minutes / Skill: simple

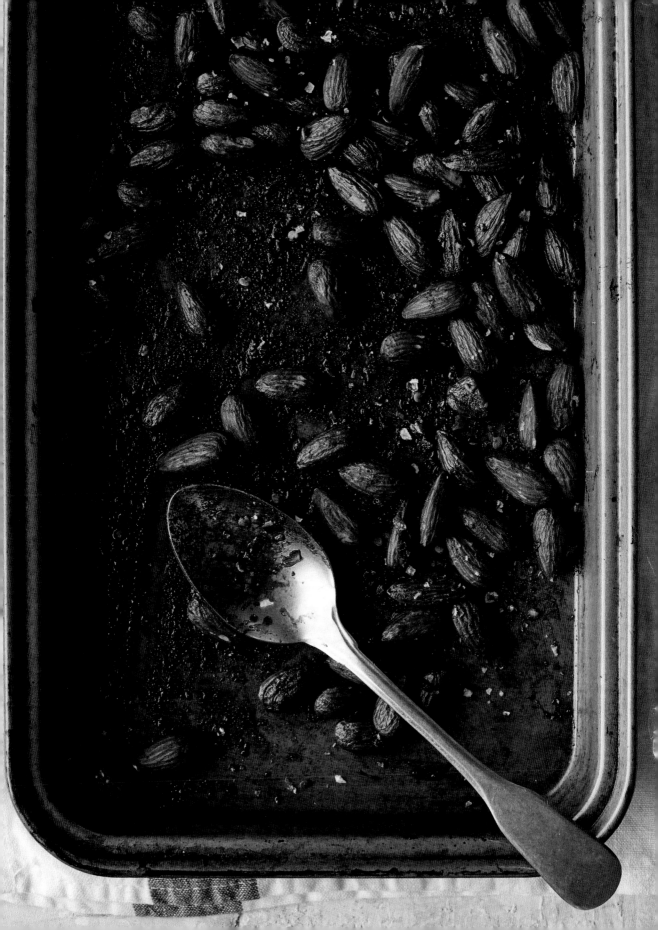

COFFEE & CHOCOLATE BITES

MAKES 10

150g porridge oats
75g ground flaxseed
2 tbsp freshly ground
    coffee beans
75g almond butter
2 tbsp runny honey
50g dried cranberries
50g chocolate chips

Energy (kCal) 200/serving	
Fat (g) 10	Fibre (g) 4
Sat fat (g) 2	Protein (g) 6
Carbs (g) 20	Salt (g) 0
Sugar (g) 9.5	

1 Combine the oats, flaxseed and coffee together in a large bowl.

2 Place the almond butter, honey and cranberries in a saucepan and warm over a low heat. When the honey and almond butter have melted, pour the mixture over the oats, add the chocolate chips and mix together.

3 Roll the mixture into 10 small balls, place on a plate and chill for 30 minutes before serving.

Prep: 10 minutes + 30 minutes chilling / Skill: simple

SEEDED FLAPJACKS

MAKES 8

140g muscovado sugar
3 tbsp maple syrup
140g butter
250g porridge oats
90g sultanas
90g mixed chopped nuts
50g dried apricots
50g mixed seeds
25g dried cranberries

Energy (kCal) 505/serving	
Fat (g) 26	Fibre (g) 4
Sat fat (g) 11	Protein (g) 9
Carbs (g) 58	Salt (g) 0.3
Sugar (g) 35	

1 Preheat the oven to 160°C/Fan 140°C/Gas 3. Line a baking tray with baking parchment.

2 Put the sugar, maple syrup and butter in a medium saucepan over a medium heat. When the butter has melted and the sugar has dissolved, pour the mixture into a large heatproof bowl. Add the remaining ingredients and mix well.

3 Pour the mixture into the prepared tray, then press down with the back of a spoon to form an even layer.

4 Bake for 30 minutes. Allow to cool before cutting into 8 bars.

Prep: 10 minutes / Cook: 30 minutes / Skill: simple

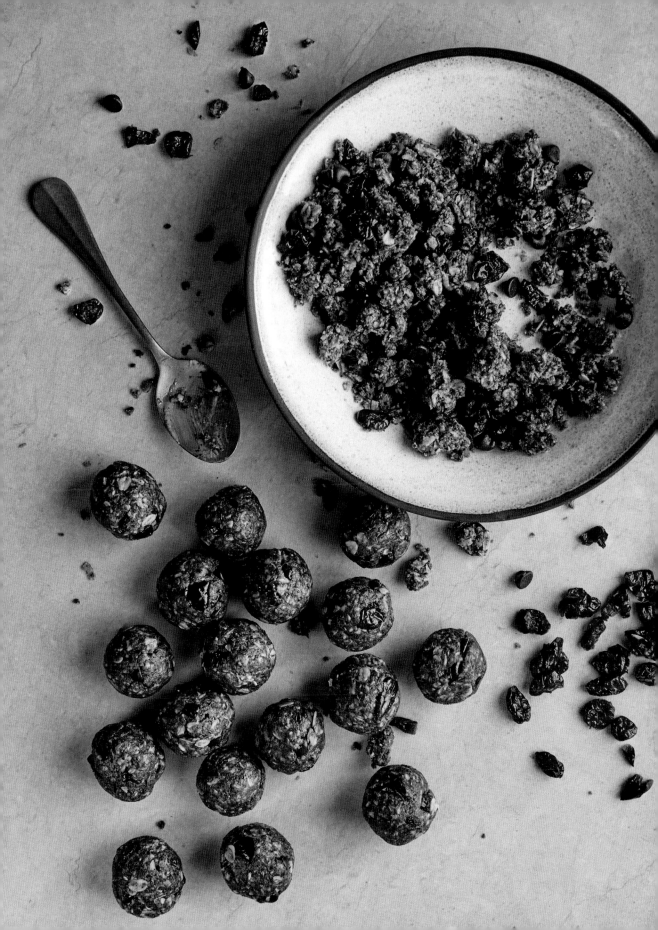

MASCARPONE CHOCOLATE MOUSSE

SERVES 2

120g mascarpone cheese
1 tbsp cocoa powder
2 tsp runny honey

Energy (kCal) 312/serving	
Fat (g) 28	Fibre (g) 0
Sat fat (g) 18.5	Protein (g) 4.5
Carbs (g) 9	Salt (g) 0.1
Sugar (g) 8	

1 Mix all the ingredients together in a large bowl. Spoon into 2 ramekins and chill in the fridge for 30 minutes or more before serving.

Prep: 5 minutes / Skill: simple

MINI CRUSTLESS AVOCADO & CHILLI QUICHES

MAKES 6

4 eggs
¼ ripe avocado, diced
6 cherry tomatoes, chopped
¼ red chilli, finely chopped
salt and pepper

Energy (kCal) 368/serving	
Fat (g) 31	Fibre (g) 1
Sat fat (g) 15	Protein (g) 9
Carbs (g) 13	Salt (g) 0.2
Sugar (g) 12	

1 Preheat the oven to 180°C/Fan 160°C/Gas 4. Line 6 muffin tray cups with paper cases.

2 Crack the eggs into a bowl, season with salt and pepper and whisk well. Add the avocado, tomatoes and chilli and mix again.

3 Divide the mixture equally between the paper cases and bake for 8–9 minutes. Allow to cool slightly before serving.

Prep: 10 minutes / Cook: 8–9 minutes / Skill: simple

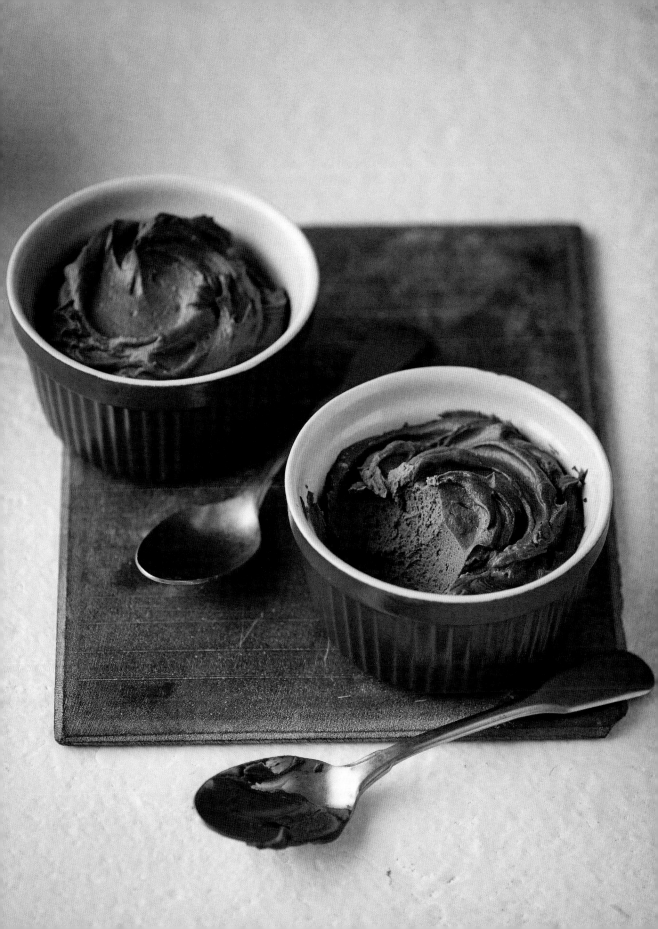

SPINACH & FETA HUMMUS WITH CRUDITÉS

SERVES 2

1 x 400g tin chickpeas, drained
3 handfuls of baby spinach
    leaves
50g feta cheese
2 garlic cloves
1 tsp ground cumin
2 tsp tahini
3 tbsp olive oil
salt and pepper

For the crudités

selection of vegetables
    for dipping, e.g. carrot,
    cucumber, pepper,
    broccoli, cauliflower

1 Place all the ingredients for the hummus in a food processor and blend until smooth. Adjust the seasoning as necessary.

2 Cut your chosen vegetables into batons and enjoy with your hummus.

Prep: 10 minutes / Skill: simple

Energy (kCal) 160/serving	
Fat (g) 10.5	Fibre (g) 5
Sat fat (g) 1.5	Protein (g) 6
Carbs (g) 8	Salt (g) 0.1
Sugar (g) 0	

PEANUT BUTTER ENERGY BALLS

MAKES 8

120g peanut butter
60g ground almonds
3 tbsp maple syrup
pinch of salt

1 Put all the ingredients into a bowl and stir until combined.

2 Divide the mixture into 8 equal pieces, then roll each one into a ball. Place on a plate and chill for 30 minutes before eating.

Prep: 5 minutes + 30 minutes chilling / Skill: simple

Energy (kCal) 162/serving	
Fat (g) 12	Fibre (g) 1
Sat fat (g) 2	Protein (g) 6
Carbs (g) 7	Salt (g) 0.3
Sugar (g) 5.5	

CHOCOLATE BROWNIES

MAKES 8

150g unsweetened dark
  chocolate, broken into pieces
150g unsalted butter, chopped
4 large eggs
90g Truvia (sugar-free
  sweetener)
90g ground almonds
30g cocoa powder
½ tsp baking powder

Energy (kCal) 368/serving	
Fat (g) 31	Fibre (g) 1
Sat fat (g) 15	Protein (g) 9
Carbs (g) 13	Salt (g) 0.2
Sugar (g) 12	

1 Preheat the oven to 190°C/Fan 170°C/Gas 5.
Line a baking tray with baking parchment.

2 Place a heatproof bowl over a pan of simmering water;
it should not actually touch the water. Put the chocolate
and butter in the bowl and allow to melt. Once melted,
stir together, then remove from the heat and set aside
to cool slightly.

3 Put the eggs and Truvia into another bowl and whisk
until pale. Gradually pour the egg mixture into the
chocolate, stirring constantly as you do so.

4 Combine the almonds, cocoa powder and baking
powder in another bowl. Add to the chocolate mixture,
off the heat, and gently fold together.

5 Pour the brownie mixture into the prepared tray,
then bake for 15 minutes. Allow to cool before slicing
into squares.

Prep: 20 minutes / Cook: 15 minutes / Skill: simple

PROTEIN SMOOTHIES

All the following shake recipes serve one and take about two minutes to make. In each case, prepare all the ingredients as directed, then whizz in a blender. Pour into a glass and enjoy. Make sure you check the macros of these shakes as some have large amounts of carbs in them.

SPINACH & FLAXSEED PROTEIN SHAKE

handful of baby spinach
½ mango, peeled and stoned
1 ripe banana
1 tbsp flaxseed or linseed
1 scoop protein powder
1 tbsp chia seeds
350ml almond milk

Energy (kCal) 384/serving	
Fat (g) 16	Fibre (g) 16
Sat fat (g) 2.5	Protein (g) 29
Carbs (g) 56	Salt (g) 0.5
Sugar (g) 47	

SUPER-GREEN PROTEIN SHAKE

250ml almond milk
1 scoop protein powder
handful of baby spinach leaves
1 kiwi fruit, peeled
2 kale leaves, stalks removed
1 tsp runny honey
1 ripe banana

Energy (kCal) 293/serving	
Fat (g) 5	Fibre (g) 3.5
Sat fat (g) 0.8	Protein (g) 22.5
Carbs (g) 38.5	Salt (g) 0
Sugar (g) 36	

MIXED BERRY PROTEIN SHAKE

1 ripe banana
150g fresh or frozen mixed berries
1 scoop protein powder
300ml water
1 tbsp runny honey

Energy (kCal) 285/serving	
Fat (g) 2	Fibre (g) 6
Sat fat (g) 0.8	Protein (g) 21
Carbs (g) 43	Salt (g) 0
Sugar (g) 41	

CINNAMON, BANANA & OAT PROTEIN SHAKE

1 ripe banana
25g porridge oats
2 tbsp Greek yoghurt
½ tsp ground cinnamon
1 tsp runny honey
1 scoop protein powder
250ml semi-skimmed milk

Energy (kCal) 451/serving	
Fat (g) 10.5	Fibre (g) 3.5
Sat fat (g) 6	Protein (g) 33
Carbs (g) 54.5	Salt (g) 0.3
Sugar (g) 35.5	

BLUEBERRY & ALMOND BUTTER PROTEIN SHAKE

150g blueberries
1 scoop protein powder
1 tbsp almond butter
1 tbsp chia seeds
250ml almond milk

Energy (kCal) 395/serving	
Fat (g) 17	Fibre (g) 10
Sat fat (g) 2	Protein (g) 27
Carbs (g) 28	Salt (g) 0
Sugar (g) 21	

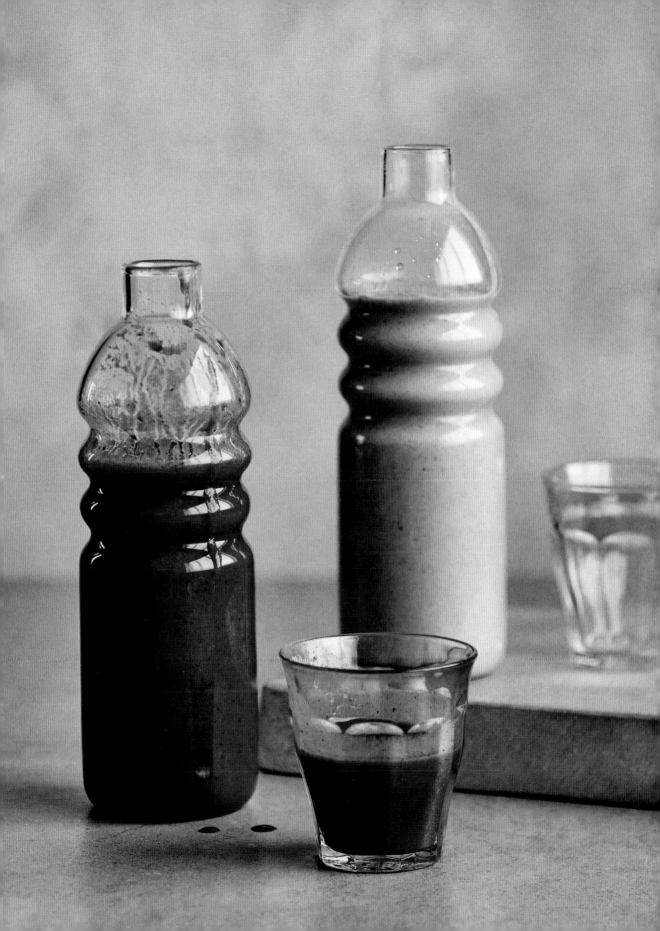

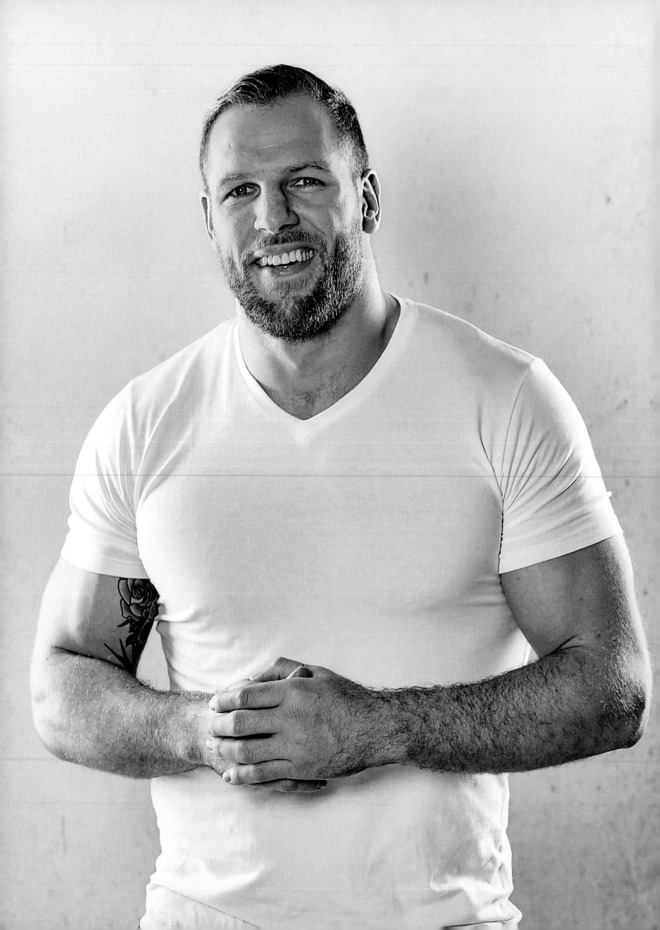

Chapter 8
FAQs

Here is a selection of questions and answers that often crop up via my website and social media sites.

Is *Perfect Fit* for beginners?

Yes. It covers everything you need to know, even if you have never trained before. Anything that I publish on my website is clearly divided into manageable chunks that work for any ability, and the same is true of this book. I have created an 8-week plan specifically for beginners and designed to get you used to training. However, it will also be useful to those who already some training experience, helping you build up to the 12-week plan and thus to get better results. Advanced users will really find something to test themselves.

Can women use *Perfect Fit*?

Absolutely. Any women who want to get into shape and make some changes to their body will find the answers in this book. **Perfect Fit is totally unisex** because there is just no need to distinguish between what men and women do in regard to training and diet. Many fitness programmes pretend otherwise, but that's a marketing ploy. *Perfect Fit* will get women great results, and you won't end up looking 'bulky'.

Can young people do this programme?

Opinions differ as to when youngsters should start lifting weights, but I started when I was 16, so of course teenagers can use this plan. Just make sure you do it under supervision, and always seek advice on technique. If you want to learn, download my introduction to rugby fitness (www.jameshaskell.com/products/training-ebooks) to get all the starting advice you could ever want.

What if I am a beginner to lifting weights?

The main part of this programme is tough and based on lifting weights, so if you have never picked up a weight before, I recommend you seek professional advice to take you through the basics. All the sessions in the programme are explained in minute detail, with pictures to back them up. You might find it helpful to repeat the beginner's 8-week programme a few times to build up your knowledge and technique before moving on to the full 12-week plan. The training chapter contains suggestions about how best to follow the programme if you find it a struggle (see page 30).

Can I move the training programme around?

In general, I recommend you stick to the order in which I've arranged the programme, but it is possible to move certain parts around, e.g. leg weights and upper body days. **If you do swap sessions around, make sure you don't do the same body part two days in a row.** What you cannot do is to take sessions out or remove rest days. You can move rest days around if necessary, but you must keep the same number of them. The programmes give you two rest days a week, with one being an optional training day. You must always take one day off.

If you find something particularly hard, you can adapt the exercise or stick with it until you get better. This programme is not about doing the things you like or want to do; the idea is to follow it to the letter.

What happens if I get injured or ill?

Injury and illness happen to us all. Make sure you note where you are in the programme and go back to that point when you are able to perform again. Try not to train when ill or injured, as that can prolong both. Do not worry if you miss sessions. The most important thing is to keep your nutrition on track as that will ensure you won't lose too much time.

If you have an injury to a certain area but are otherwise fit, you can adapt the sessions to avoid that area and keep making progress.

This book includes lots of advice about how to deal with injury and how to recover (see pages 177–188). There are also some tips about supplements you can take to help boost your immune system (see page 213).

Can I eat out while training?

Of course you can, but you will need to make sure you do it within your allotted macros. I know this is not always possible, but most of the time it is achievable, especially if you use the app MyFitnessPal. Do not expect to eat out often, though, particularly if you are looking to lose weight and body fat. However, life is for living, and if you want to change things up now and then, just factor it in and don't let it derail your progress.

Do I have to take supplements?

No. Among the suggested protocols for getting the best results out of this programme (see page 30), some specific supplements are recommended for certain situations. However, a good diet should supply what you need and should always be your first port of call. That is why this book includes extensive information about nutrition and a chapter of fantastic recipes.

Any advice for vegetarians and vegans?

You can still follow this programme if you are not a meat eater, but I recommend that you seek professional nutrition advice. I simply don't know enough about being a vegan or vegetarian to fully advise you. What I do know is that it's perfectly possible for anyone to create a good nutrition plan even within certain limitations. The key thing is to understand what foods you can eat to fulfil your macros.

Can I use this training programme during the season?

Lots of rugby players follow this plan and often ask this question. For two reasons, I suggest you do not use the muscle-building part of the programme while competing in any sports season. First, you will get supersore from this type of training. Second, it is unhelpful to be in a size-building phase while trying to perform. The best time to do this programme is pre-season or off-season. However, you can use the fat-loss sessions during your normal training week, and add one of the resistance sessions as well. You might need to adjust the rest periods and number of sets.

Can I do the programme if I am not a member of a gym?

Yes, you can. The 8-week programme can be done at home and is designed specifically for non-gym users. For the full 12-week programme, though, you will need access to free weights and machines. Of course, the 12-week plan does include sessions you can do without a gym, but if you want to get amazing results, you will need access to a gym.

Why are there no suggested weights for each exercise?

Simply because everyone following *Perfect Fit* is in different condition. There is plenty of advice within the book to help you choose the right weight and to know when you've got it wrong.

What happens if I go over my daily macros?

First, it's not the end of the world, but it must not become a daily occurrence. If you go over on one macro, you should drop the others so that your total daily calories remain the same. Everything will balance in the end, and this is particularly important if you are trying to lose weight and bodyfat. Going over your total calories is more of an issue. If it happens make sure you get back on track the next day.

If, on the other hand, you are trying to gain size and aren't too worried about extra body fat, just accept the fact you have gone over and crack on.

Can I substitute exercises?

If you find some exercises too hard, you need to modify what you are doing and take things back a progression. In the case of movements that cause you discomfort or pain, find a similar movement or exercise that doesn't produce those symptoms.

Many exercises in *Perfect Fit* can be modified to bodyweight work, which is less arduous than weighted work, very good for beginners, and useful if you have limited equipment to hand, perhaps when you are on holiday. In this case, you can use bands and dumbbells if you don't have access to a fully stocked gym.

Can I eat cheat meals?

If you fall off the nutrition wagon and end up having a cheat meal, it's not a disaster and won't destroy your progress. The important thing is to get back onto your nutritional plan for the meals that follow the 'blip' because more than one day of poor eating will really mess up all the progress you have made.

The fact of the matter is that you are trying to make drastic changes to your body, so eating poorly is not an option. However, I do understand that we are all human and sometimes the urge to break out is too strong to resist. If you simply must have a bad meal, hold out for as long as you can and do it towards the end of the programme. You should only 'reward' yourself when the job is done, and try to keep it to just one meal then get back on track.

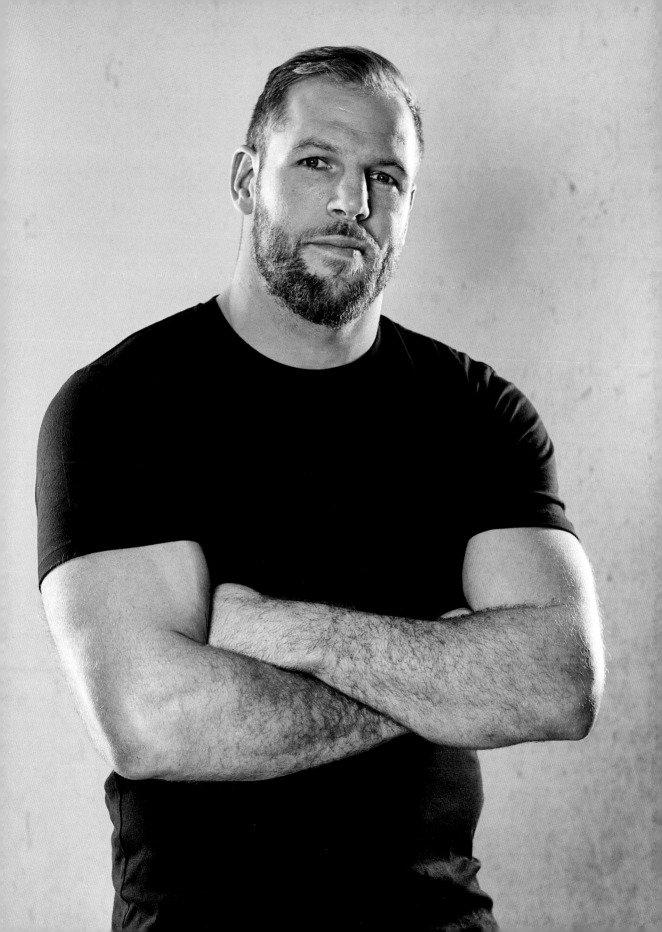

ACKNOWLEDGEMENTS

It's really a no brainer who I have to thank first in helping me put *Perfect Fit* together. My long-suffering agent, Clare Hulton, who has gone above and beyond in the line of duty. Thank you for always being on the end of the phone and ready to step in to fix any issues. You are a literary super-hero and would make a great UN peacekeeper.

To my amazing girlfriend, Chloe, who kept my head from rolling off my shoulders day in, day out. You kept me fed and watered through the whole process, and without your amazing support I could not have done this. Thank you for reading my words, steering me in the right direction and showing me the way of healthy eating.

To my Mum and Dad for always pushing me to do these things and giving me the support I need. To my Dad especially for helping get me a book deal in the first place – adding value as you always do.

To Omar Meziane – chef extraordinaire – thank you for all your amazing recipes and taking the time to sit down and turn my ramblings into tasty meals. You are a genius in the kitchen and have kept many sports people happy with your skills.

I want to thank Fiona Hunter for all her time and effort checking through my nutritional work, correcting my mistakes and helping me out last minute, or whenever I called her up in a panic.

I have known Matt Lovell for many years; he was the first guy to help me with my nutrition and taught me so much. Thank you for taking the time to read my book in the early days.

Thank you to Jake Saunders from Pulse who not only sorted out a location for the exercise photos, but also featured in most of them, saved the day and convinced Pulse to supply all the gym equipment.

Thank you to Kirby Young for volunteering to appear in the book as my female model. You gave up your time and for that I will always be grateful.